ECG 🐮 STAMPEDE

First Edition

Authors

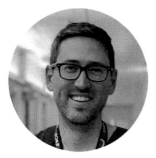

Benjamin L. Cooper, MD, MEd, FACEP

Dr. Cooper is a board-certified emergency medicine physician and assistant professor at McGovern Medical School at the University of Texas Health Science Center at Houston (UTHealth) where he serves as the associate residency program director and co-director of the emergency medicine medical education fellowship.

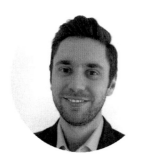

Jonathan A. Giordano, DO, MS, MEd

Dr. Giordano is a board-certified emergency medicine physician and assistant professor at McGovern Medical School at the University of Texas Health Science Center at Houston (UTHealth) where he serves as the director of undergraduate medical education and co-director of the emergency medicine medical education fellowship.

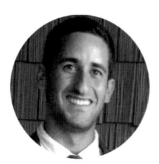

Tom T. Fadial, MD

Dr. Fadial is a board-certified emergency medicine physician and assistant professor at McGovern Medical School at the University of Texas Health Science Center at Houston (UTHealth) where he serves as the Education Technology and Innovation Officer for the department of emergency medicine. He is also the creator of ddxof.com, where there's an algorithm for the evaluation and management of just about every chief complaint.

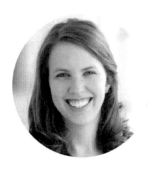

Catherine E. Reynolds, MD

Dr. Reynolds is a board-certified emergency medicine physician and assistant professor at McGovern Medical School at the University of Texas Health Science Center at Houston (UTHealth) where she serves as the clerkship director for emergency medicine.

Acknowledgements

We would like to acknowledge those who played a significant role in the development of this curriculum. Thank you to Dr. Yashwant Chathampally for your expert content review during ECG Stampede's infancy. Thank you to Dr. Daniel Ostermayer for your creative and publishing expertise. Thank you to the emergency medicine residents of McGovern Medical School at UTHealth; without you, this would not exist.

Dedicated to Micah and Jonah:
You color every beat.

Preface: How to Use This Book

This book started as a series of lectures given to the emergency medicine residents of McGovern Medical School at UTHealth in Houston, TX. Over several years, it evolved into an entire curriculum with companion videos (**ecgstampede.com**).

You will note that the book is divided into sections designated as units instead of chapters. This book is a curriculum in electrocardiography triage, meant to be taken as a whole, not necessarily to be used as a reference (although it can be). Concepts are interleaved, or spaced out, throughout ten units, making it difficult to select them out. For example, you'll find several units that touch on conduction disturbances, not just one chapter. Each unit is comprised of five to nine cases and each case starts out with a narrative prompt (e.g. "39 yo F p/w chest pain" – 39 year-old female presents with chest pain), an electrocardiogram (ECG), blank spaces for standardized interpretation, and one or more thought-provoking question(s). It is our intention for the reader to attempt to interpret each ECG and to answer the corresponding questions prior to turning the page and reading the answer. We understand this may seem tedious, repetitive, and frustrating at times when you don't know the answer, but we believe learning happens during that struggle. We think this is the best way to learn electrocardiography.

Also, if you're interested in practicing your skills on the fly, feel free to visit **ecgstampede.com** for a fun, interactive experience in ECG triage. There's an ECG Stampede application that can be downloaded in the Apple and Google Play stores. We invite you to be one of thousands to have downloaded and enjoyed the experience.

Thank you for your purchase of this book and we welcome your feedback. Please feel free to contact me with any comments or suggestions.

Ben
ben@ecgstampede.com

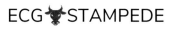
Table of Contents

Unit 1

Systematic Approach to ECG Interpretation
Anatomic Distribution
Conduction Disturbances
Ventricular Preexcitation

#1 – 39 yo F p/w chest pain

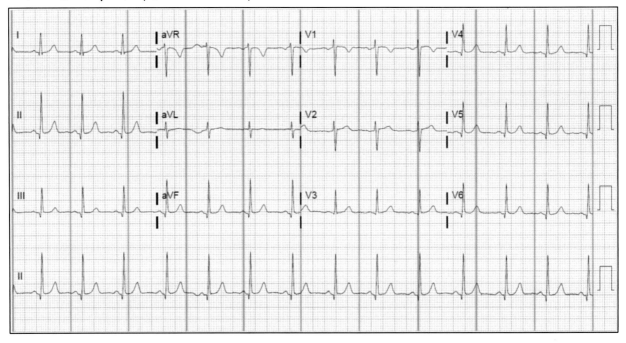

Rate: _____ Rhythm: _____ Axis: _____ Intervals: _____ Ischemia: _____

Describe the systematic approach to electrocardiography (ECG) interpretation.

#1 – 39 yo F p/w chest pain

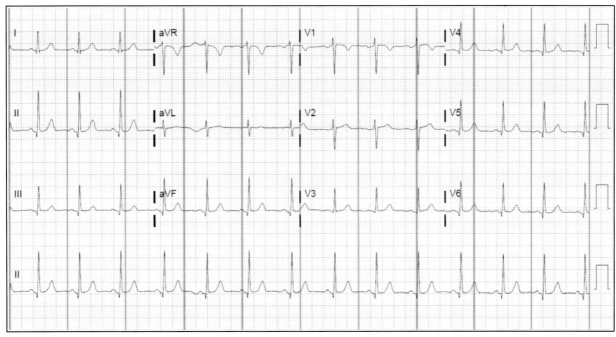

Systematic approach to ECG interpretation

Rate: 84   Rhythm: sinus   Axis: normal   Intervals: normal   Ischemia: none

Rate

To determine the rate, count the number of large boxes between QRS complexes and divide 300 by that number. This works because each small box is 40 ms and each large box is 200 ms (or five small boxes); therefore, one beat per 200 ms equates to 300 bpm, one beat per 400 ms equates to 150 bpm, etc. The rate can be determined quickly by memorizing this series of numbers as you count the number of large boxes between complexes: 300, 150, 100, 75, 60, 50, 43. At slower rates, it may be easier to count the total number of complexes along the entire rhythm strip and multiply by six (since the ECG represents ten seconds).

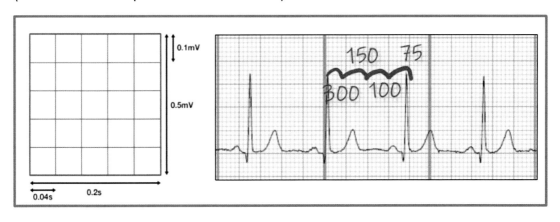

Rhythm

We'll be reviewing rhythm as we progress in the curriculum. For now, suffice it to say that if there is a P wave for every QRS, and a QRS for every P wave, the rhythm is likely to be sinus – that is, arising from the sinus node in the right atrium and progressing normally through the conduction system to generate ventricular depolarization.

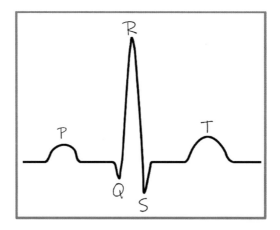

P wave, atrial depolarization; QRS, ventricular depolarization; T wave, ventricular repolarization.

Axis

Axis is the term used to describe the direction of the resultant vector of ventricular depolarization. Normally, the ventricles will depolarize from the superior septum towards the apex, resulting in a depolarization vector that is projected near the same direction as lead II (60 degrees below the horizontal). The axis can be determined observing the direction of QRS deflection in leads I and aVF as depicted below.

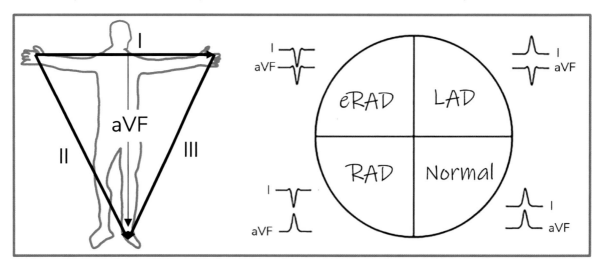

LAD, left axis deviation; RAD, right axis deviation; eRAD, extreme right axis deviation

Intervals

We will focus on three intervals: the PR interval, the QRS width, and the QT interval. The PR interval starts at the initial deflection of the P wave and ends at the initial deflection of the QRS complex. The QT interval begins at the initial deflection of the QRS complex and ends at the end of the T wave. The QRS width begins at the initial deflection of the QRS complex and ends at the J point (the intersection between the S wave and the ST segment).

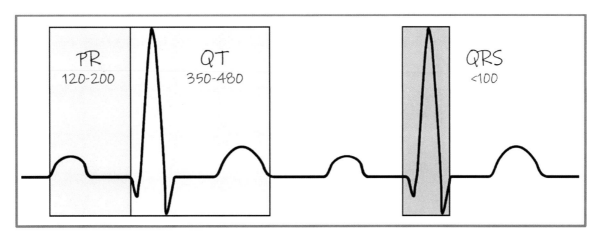

PR interval, QT interval, and QRS width shown with normal ranges in ms.

Signs of Ischemia

Finally, once the rate, rhythm, axis, and intervals have been determined, then look for signs of ischemia. Potential signs of ischemia include hyperacute T waves, T wave inversions, ST deviations (elevation or depression), and Q waves.

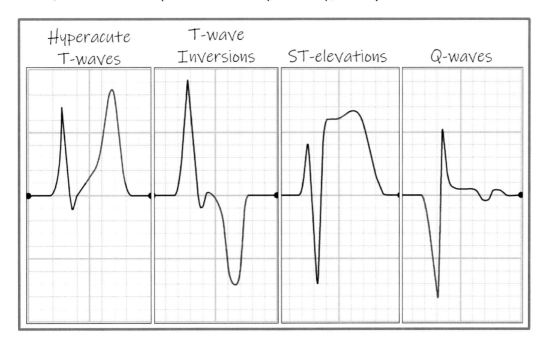

#2 – 50 yo M p/w chest pain

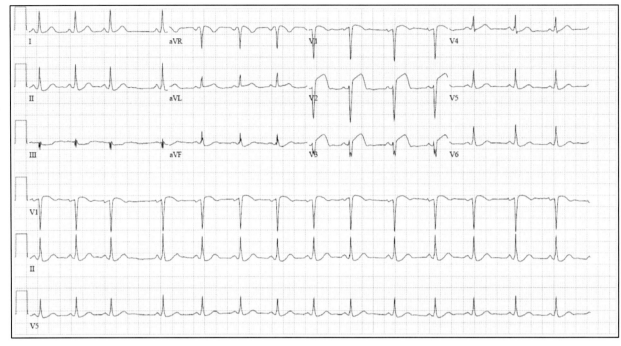

Rate: _____ Rhythm: _____ Axis: _____ Intervals: _____ Ischemia: _____

What are the critical actions?

What complications should you expect/anticipate?

Complete the following table.

DISTRIBUTION	CORONARY ARTERY	LEADS	RECIPROCAL CHANGES
1. Inferior			
2. Lateral			
3. Anterior			
4. Posterior			

#2 – 50 yo M p/w chest pain

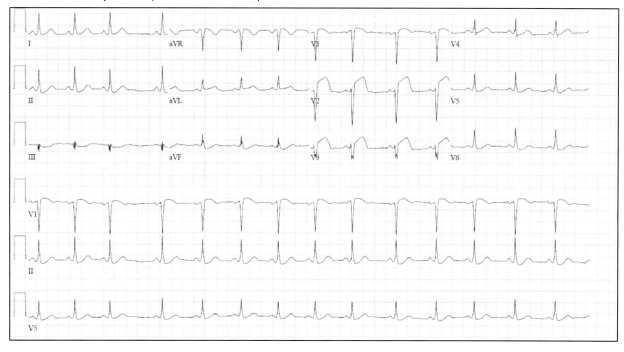

Anterior STEMI

Rate: 84 Rhythm: sinus Axis: normal Intervals: normal Ischemia: STE V1-3 with reciprocal changes in inferolateral leads

What are the critical actions?

The initial critical actions include securing intravenous access, delivering oxygen as needed, placing the patient on the monitor with defibrillation pads, administering sublingual and/or intravenous nitroglycerin for pain relief, non-enteric coated aspirin, +/- P2Y12 inhibitors, +/- heparin gtt, and thrombolytics if transfer time greater than 120 min is anticipated.[1] While all these actions are important, nothing should delay emergent reperfusion via percutaneous coronary intervention if available, or thrombolytics if not.

What complications should you expect/anticipate?

Anterior ST-elevation myocardial infarctions (STEMIs) are large-territory infarcts. The anterior wall is responsible for a majority of the cardiac output. Complications include dysrhythmias, acute heart failure, ruptured chordae tendineae/papillary muscle, and conduction disturbances.[1]

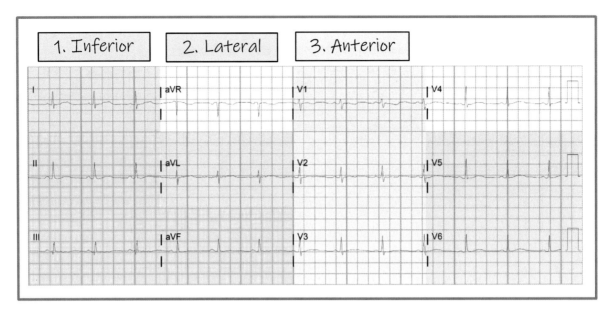

Anatomic distribution of the 12-lead ECG.

DISTRIBUTION[2,3]	CORONARY ARTERY	LEADS	RECIPROCAL CHANGES
1. Inferior	RCA, PDA	II, III, aVF	Anterior, High Lateral
2. Lateral	LCx*	I, aVL, V5, V6	Inferior*
3. Anterior	LAD	V1-V6	Inferior, Posterior
4. Posterior	RCA, LCx	Posterior	Anterior (esp. V1)

*In left dominant hearts, a LCx occlusion can involve both lateral and inferior walls simultaneously. RCA, right coronary artery; PDA, posterior descending artery; LCx, left circumflex artery; LAD, left anterior descending artery. Posterior infarctions will show ST depressions in the anterior distribution (see Unit 2, case #2).

#3 – 77 yo M p/w dyspnea

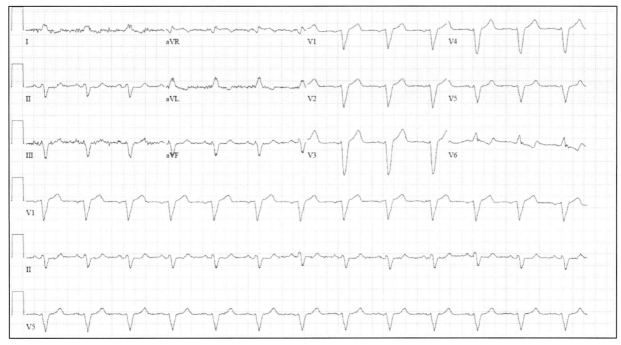

Rate: _____ Rhythm: _____ Axis: _____ Intervals: _____ Ischemia: _____

Describe the trifascicular framework of the intraventricular conduction system.

Why is the QRS complex wide?

What are the electrocardiographic criteria for making this diagnosis?

What rule can help diagnose acute myocardial infarction with an ECG like this?

#3 – 77 yo M p/w dyspnea

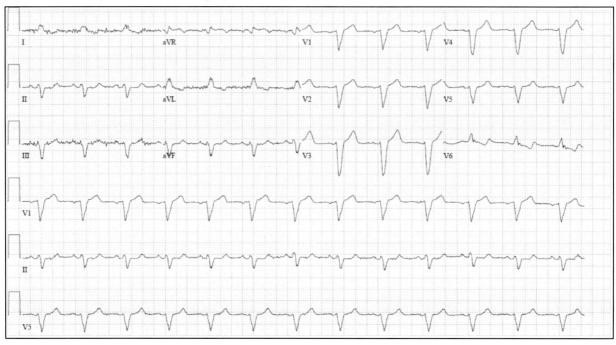

Left bundle branch block

Rate: 78 Rhythm: sinus Axis: left axis deviation Intervals: wide QRS Ischemia: none

Describe the trifascicular framework of the intraventricular conduction system.

Our current understanding of the intraventricular conduction system comes from a series of seminal papers by Rosenbaum et al from 1969 to 1973. These works elucidated three conduction terminals known as the trifascicular conduction system – one in the right ventricle (i.e. the right bundle) and two in the left ventricle (i.e. the anterior and posterior divisions of the left bundle).[4–6]

Why is the QRS complex wide?

This patient has a left bundle branch block (LBBB), which occurs when the left bundle no longer conducts, and the signal must pass to the left ventricle via myocyte-to-myocyte conduction. This pattern of conduction is slower than via the specialized conduction system, and results in a wide QRS complex (>120 ms). Conduction disturbances, like bundle branch blocks, result from structural abnormalities of the His-Purkinje system caused by necrosis, fibrosis, calcification, infiltrative disease, electrolyte disturbances, or impaired vascular supply.[7] When conduction is impaired to both left ventricular terminals (the left anterior and posterior fascicles), the result is a LBBB.

What are the electrocardiographic criteria for making this diagnosis?

The criteria are: QRS >120 ms, dominant S wave in V1, broad monophasic or notched R wave in lateral leads (I, aVL, V5, V6), +/- left axis deviation.[7-9]

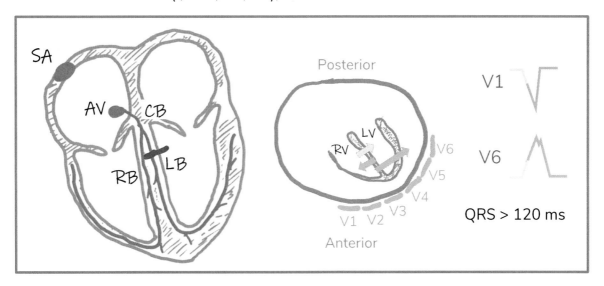

Depiction of depolarization in left bundle branch block. The septum first depolarizes from right to left (blue arrow) followed by near simultaneous depolarization of the right and left ventricles (pink arrows). The resultant vector leads to a negative deflection in V1 and a positive deflection in V6. SA, sinoatrial node; AV, atrioventricular node; RB, right bundle; LB, left bundle; CB, common bundle or junction; RV, right ventricle; LV, left ventricle; red dash represents a block of the left bundle

What rule(s) can help diagnose acute myocardial infarction with an ECG like this?

The Sgarbossa criteria, or modified Sgarbossa criteria, can help diagnose acute myocardial infraction in the presence of LBBB.[10,11] Concordance describes ST changes in the same direction as the QRS complex and is a powerful predictor of STEMI in the symptomatic LBBB – it is an indication for emergent reperfusion.[12] The modified Sgarbossa criteria are:

1) Concordant ST elevation of ≥ 1 mm
2) Concordant ST depression of ≥ 1 mm in V1, V2, or V3, or
3) Excessively discordant ST elevation defined as the ST/S ratio greater than 0.25.

The modified criteria are more sensitive and specific than the original criteria.[11] More recently, the Barcelona algorithm was validated.[13] For more details about the various criteria for diagnosing acute myocardial infarction in the setting of left bundle branch block, see Unit 2, case #3.

#4 – 73 yo F p/w chest pain

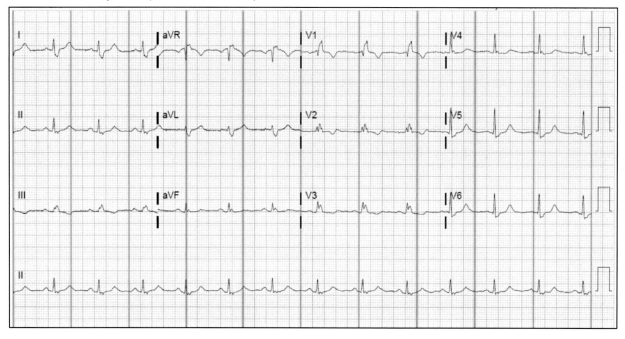

Rate: _____ Rhythm: _____ Axis: _____ Intervals: _____ Ischemia: _____

Why is the QRS complex wide?

What are the criteria for making this diagnosis?

What are the causes of it?

What ST/T changes are expected?

#4 – 73 yo F p/w chest pain

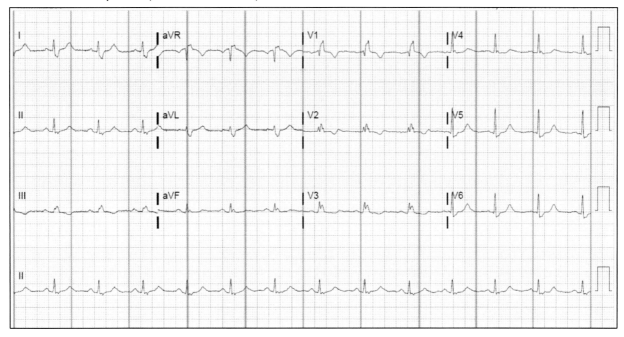

Right bundle branch block

Rate: 78 Rhythm: sinus Axis: normal Intervals: wide QRS Ischemia: none

What is the QRS complex wide?

This patient has a right bundle branch block (RBBB), which occurs when the right bundle no longer conducts, and the signal must pass to the right ventricle via myocyte-to-myocyte conduction. This pattern of conduction is slower than via the specialized conduction system, and results in a wide QRS complex (>120 ms).

What are the criteria for making this diagnosis?

The criteria are: QRS > 120 ms, RSR' pattern in V1-3 ('M-shaped'), and a wide/slurred S wave in the lateral leads (I, aVL, V5-6). Note that there is no right axis deviation associated with RBBB as there is a left axis deviation associated with left bundle branch block.[8,9]

What are the causes of it?

RBBB is common and generally not a powerful indicator of disease by itself. This is because the RBBB often has a singular blood supply as opposed to the LBBB which has a more diverse one and therefore is more consistent with significant disease. However, a new RBBB in a patient with unexplained respiratory symptoms should be viewed as right ventricular outflow obstruction until proven otherwise. RBBB can be caused by right ventricular hypertrophy/cor pulmonale, pulmonary embolism, ischemic heart disease, rheumatic heart disease, myocarditis or cardiomyopathy, degenerative disease of the conduction system, or congenital heart disease (e.g. atrial septal defect).

What ST/T changes are expected?

Expected repolarization abnormalities in the setting of RBBB include T wave inversions in V1-3 and slight discordant ST depressions. ST elevation in these leads is never normal; even slight ST elevations in V1-3 may represent STEMI.[9,12]

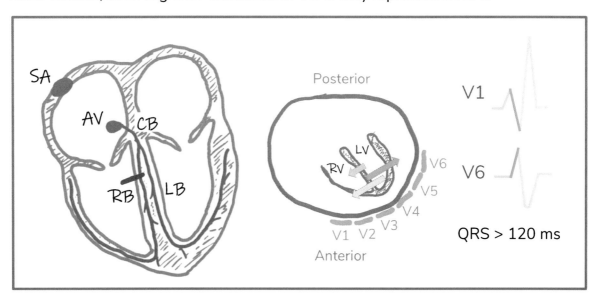

Direction of depolarization in right bundle branch block. The septum first depolarizes from left to right (blue arrow) followed by left ventricular depolarization (pink arrow) and right ventricular depolarization (green arrow). The result is an rSR' pattern in V1, and a wide S wave in the lateral leads (I, aVL, V5, V6). SA, sinoatrial node; AV, atrioventricular node; RB, right bundle; LB, left bundle; CB, common bundle or junction; RV, right ventricle; LV, left ventricle; red dash represents a block of the left bundle

#5 – 27 yo F p/w palpitations

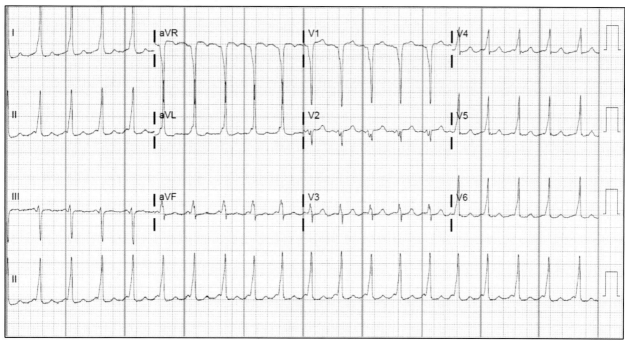

Rate: _____ Rhythm: _____ Axis: _____ Intervals: _____ Ischemia: _____

What are two interval abnormalities?

What is the diagnosis?

#5 – 27 yo F p/w palpitations

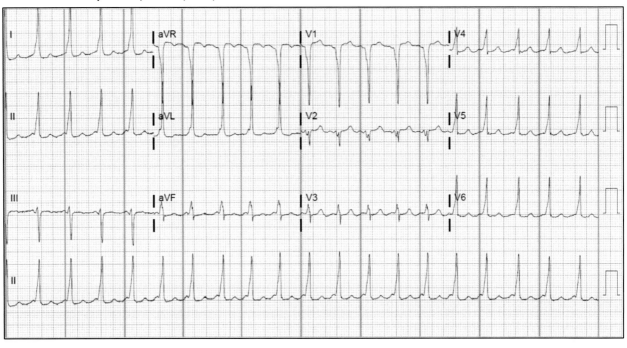

Ventricular pre-excitation

Rate: 120   Rhythm: sinus tachycardia   Axis: normal   Intervals: short PR, wide QRS
Ischemia: none

What are two interval abnormalities?

Short PR, slightly widened QRS due to slurred upstroke of the R wave referred to as a delta wave[2,14]

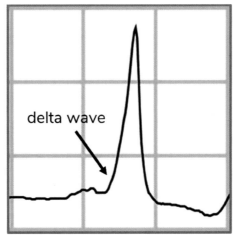

Classic triad of findings for pre-excitation: shortened PR interval, slightly widened QRS, and delta wave

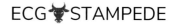

What is the diagnosis?

Pre-excitation is a condition in which an accessory pathway exists between the atria and the ventricles, often referred to as the bundle of Kent.[14] When the accessory pathway conducts in an anterograde direction, the ventricles are "pre-excited," yielding the characteristic delta wave on the ECG. Because of the accessory pathway, patients are at risk for developing antidromic (wide complex, anterograde conduction through the accessory pathway and retrograde conduction through the atrioventricular node) or orthodromic (narrow complex, anterograde conduction through the atrioventricular node and retrograde conduction through the accessory pathway) reentrant rhythms.[2,14,15] When dysrhythmias occur involving the accessory pathway, it is referred to as the Wolf-Parkinson-White syndrome (WPW). In Unit 6, we will discuss the unique circumstance of atrial fibrillation in the setting of WPW.

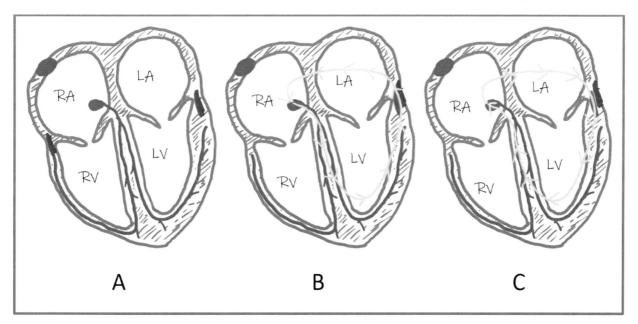

Depiction of orthodromic and antidromic atrioventricular reentrant tachycardias possible with the Wolf-Parkinson-White syndrome. The red bars in panel A represent possible locations of the accessory pathway (type A, between LA and LV; type B, between RA and RV). The blue line in panel B represents orthodromic conduction (narrow complex) and the blue line in panel C represents antidromic conduction (wide complex). RA, right atrium; RV, right ventricle; LA, left atrium; LV, left ventricle.

Unit 2

Anatomic Distributions
Conduction Disturbances

#1 – 57 yo F p/w lower extremity edema

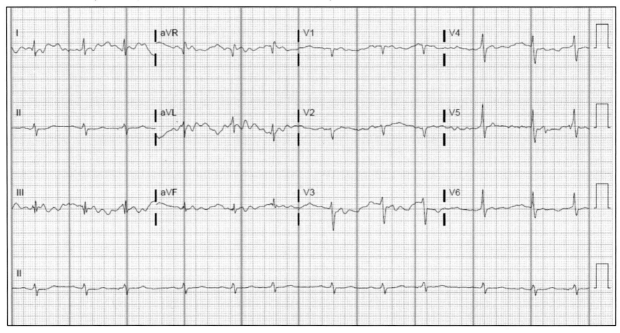

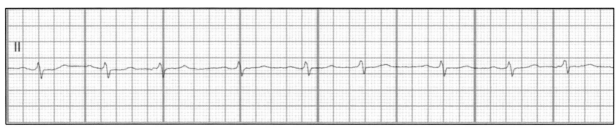

Rate: _____ Rhythm: _____ Axis: _____ Intervals: _____ Ischemia: _____

This is a rhythm case. What is the rhythm?

#1 – 57 yo F p/w lower extremity edema

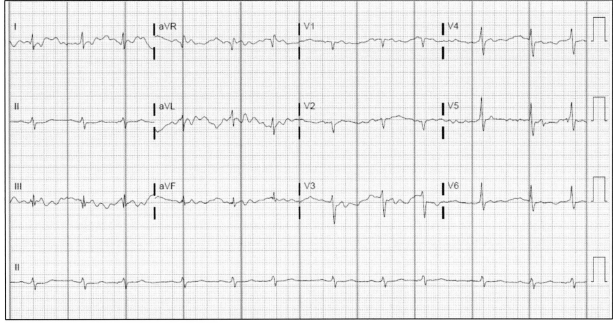

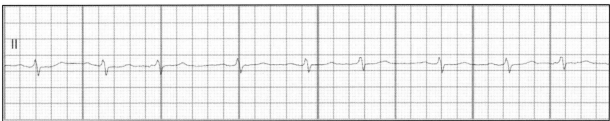

Junctional trigeminy

<u>Rate</u>: 72   <u>Rhythm</u>: Junctional trigeminy   <u>Axis</u>: normal   <u>Intervals</u>: normal   <u>Ischemia</u>: none

This is a rhythm case. What is the rhythm?

This rhythm was mistakenly called atrial fibrillation based on the computer interpretation (and eventually confirmed by the cardiologist), but the rhythm is *regularly* irregular, unlike atrial fibrillation which is *irregularly* irregular. There are two sinus beats followed by a prematurely conducted junctional complex in a pattern of trigeminy. This patient was going to be admitted for heparin, echo, and cards consult but, instead, was discharged without anticoagulation. One important part of making the correct interpretation is recognizing an artifactual baseline and repeating the ECG. Over-reliance on the computerized interpretation is a common and high-risk pitfall.

#2 – 43 yo F p/w chest pain

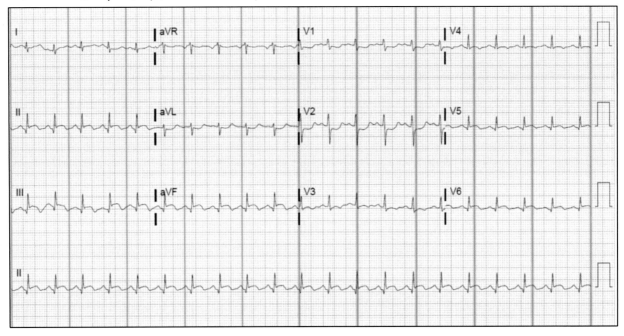

Rate: _____ Rhythm: _____ Axis: _____ Intervals: _____ Ischemia: _____

What is the anatomic distribution of this STEMI?

#2 – 43 yo F p/w chest pain

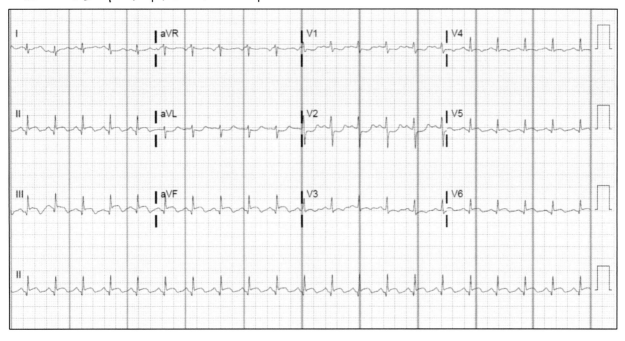

Inferior STEMI with posterior extension

Rate: 126 Rhythm: sinus tachycardia Axis: normal Intervals: normal Ischemia: inferolateral ST elevation with ST depression in V1-3 and aVL

What is the anatomic distribution of this STEMI?

This is an inferolateral STEMI with posterior extension. Features of posterior STEMI include R>S in V1-2 with "mirror" ST depression (especially horizontal or down-sloping and concave) and upright T waves. Posterior myocardial infarction is commonly confused with anterior subendocardial ischemia; however, the T waves are expected to be negatively deflected with anterior subendocardial ischemia (unless early on when they can mirror posterior hyperacute T waves). 5-10% of all myocardial infarctions are isolated posterior and not associated with inferior ST elevation. Isolated posterior myocardial infarctions are associated with longer door-to-balloon times and worse outcomes because they are frequently missed.[16,17] ST elevation of at least 0.5 mm in posterior leads can help secure the diagnosis. This patient had a total occlusion of the left circumflex and a left-dominant blood supply.

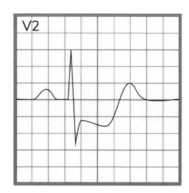

Typical anterior precordial (V1-V3) findings of posterior myocardial infarctions are R/S ratio > 1, ST depressions, and upright T waves. The appearance of tall R waves is the posterior equivalent of Q waves.

Here's an example of an ECG that shows findings consistent with a posterior myocardial infarction. This patient was found to have a complete occlusion of the second obtuse marginal branch of the left circumflex artery.

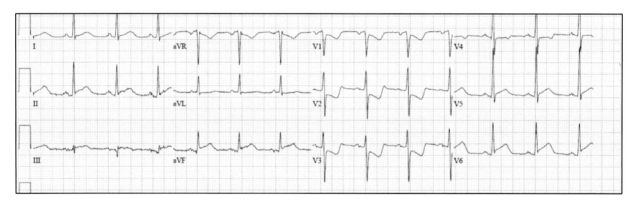

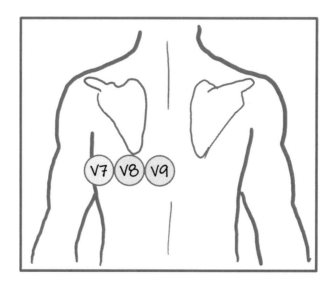

Posterior leads placed under the left scapula and designated as V7, V8, and V9.

#3 – 55 yo F p/w chest pain

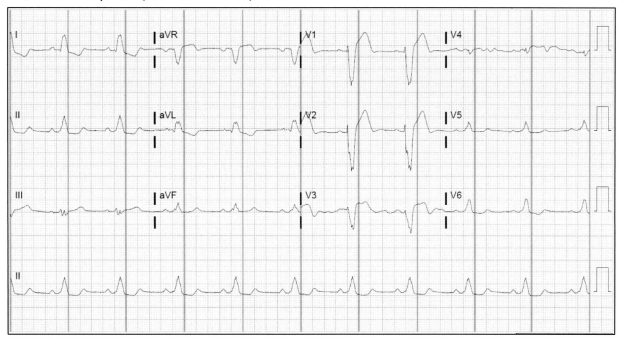

Rate: _____ Rhythm: _____ Axis: _____ Intervals: _____ Ischemia: _____

What are the criteria for left bundle branch block?

What are the expected ST/T changes associated with left bundle branch block?

What are the original Sgarbossa criteria?

What are the modified Sgarbossa criteria?

#3 – 55 yo F p/w chest pain

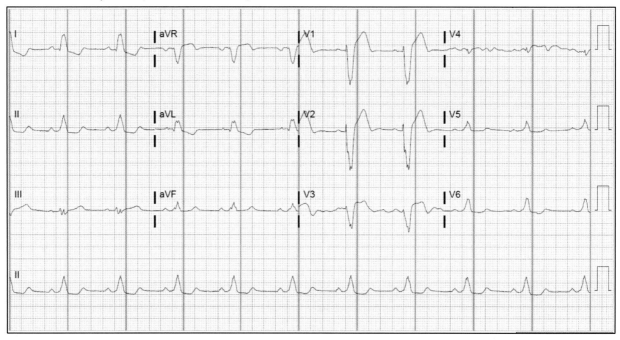

Acute myocardial infarction and left bundle branch block

Rate: 66 Rhythm: sinus Axis: normal Intervals: widened QRS Ischemia: discordant ST changes of LBBB, excessive discordance by modified Sgarbossa in V3

What are the criteria for left bundle branch block?

The criteria are: QRS >120 ms, dominant S wave in V1, broad monophasic or notched R wave in lateral leads (I, aVL, V5, V6), +/- left axis deviation.[7–9]

What are the expected ST/T changes associated with left bundle branch block?

Expected ST/T changes include discordant ST depression and T wave inversion in the lateral leads (I, aVL, V5, V6). Discordance describe ST deviation in the opposite direction of the QRS complex (i.e. ST depression in leads with up-going QRS complexes and ST elevation in leads with down-going QRS complexes).

What are the original Sgarbossa criteria?

The original Sgarbossa criteria are:

1) Concordant ST elevation ≥ 1 mm
2) Concordant ST depression ≥ 1 mm in V1, V2, or V3, or
3) Excessively discordant ST elevation (> 5 mm)

The original criteria had a weighting system for different criterion, and excessive discordance was the least specific.[10]

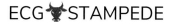

What are the modified Sgarbossa criteria?

The first two concordant criteria are the same for the modified Sgarbossa criteria, but the third criterion for excessive discordance takes the concept of proportionality into consideration – excessively discordant ST elevation is defined as an ST/S ratio greater than 0.25. The modified criteria are more sensitive and specific than the original criteria.[11] This patient met the modified criteria for excessive discordance in V3 and was found to have an occluded left anterior descending artery.

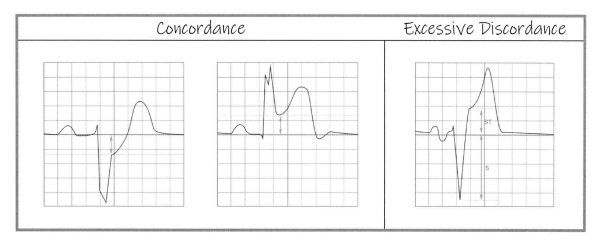

Demonstration of Sgarbossa criteria. For modified Sgarbossa criteria, the ST/S ratio should be greater than 0.25 for excessive discordance.

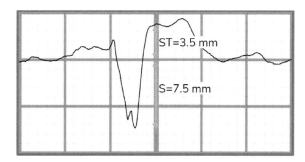

V3 complex showing the ST/S ratio of 3.5/7.5, or 0.47.

More recently, the Barcelona algorithm was validated.[13] The Barcelona algorithm differs from the modified Sgarbossa criteria in three ways: 1) While the modified Sgarbossa criteria includes concordant ST depression in only leads V1-V3, the Barcelona algorithm considers concordant ST depression in any lead; 2) the modified Sgarbossa criteria does not include excessively discordant ST depression, whereas the Barcelona criteria does; and 3) whereas the modified Sgarbossa criteria uses a quantified ratio of discordant ST elevation regardless of QRS voltage, the Barcelona algorithm applies only to leads with maximum QRS voltage of 6 mm and at least 1 mm of ST deviation (meaning a minimum ratio of 1/ 6 = 17%).[18]

#4 – 72 yo M p/w chest pain

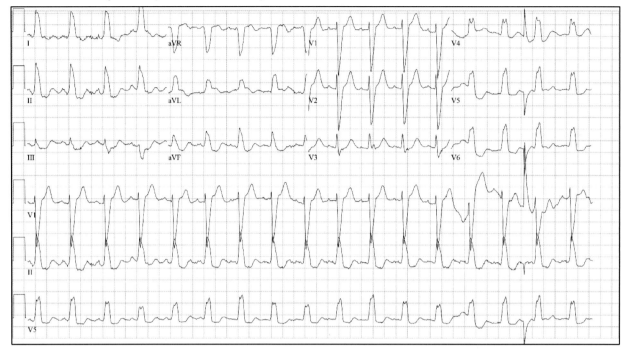

Rate: _____ Rhythm: _____ Axis: _____ Intervals: _____ Ischemia: _____

Are there any concordant ST changes?

#4 – 72 yo M p/w chest pain

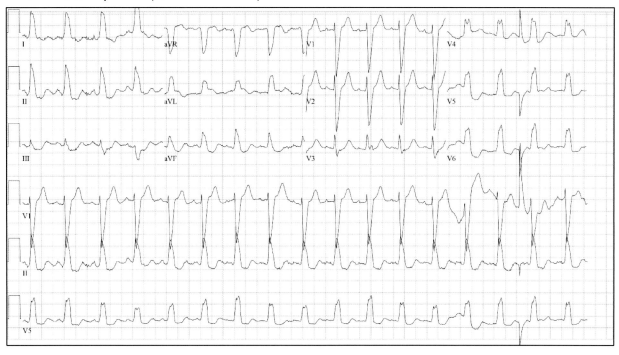

Acute myocardial infarction and left bundle branch block

Rate: 100 Rhythm: sinus Axis: normal Intervals: wide QRS Ischemia: concordance in aVL

Are there any concordant ST changes?

There is concordant ST elevation in lead aVL, suggesting acute myocardial infarction in the setting of LBBB. This patient had a total occlusion of the first diagonal branch of the left anterior descending artery.

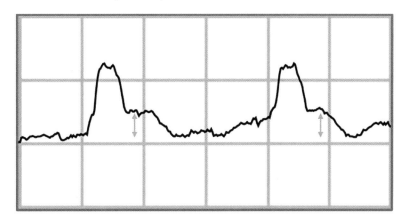

aVL complexes demonstrating greater than 1 mm of concordant ST elevation (blue lines).

#5 — 79 yo M p/w syncope

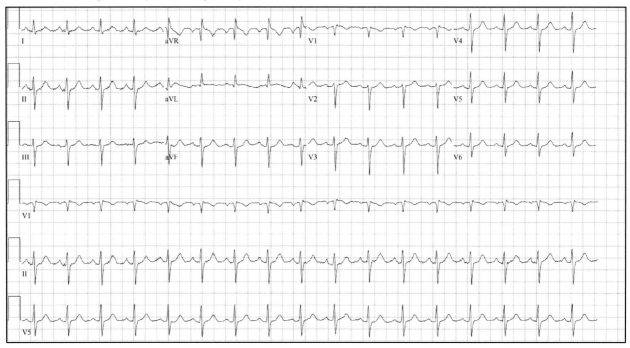

Rate: _____ Rhythm: _____ Axis: _____ Intervals: _____ Ischemia: _____

What are the five causes of left axis deviation?

What part of the conduction system is affected?

What is the significance of this finding?

#5 – 79 yo M p/w syncope

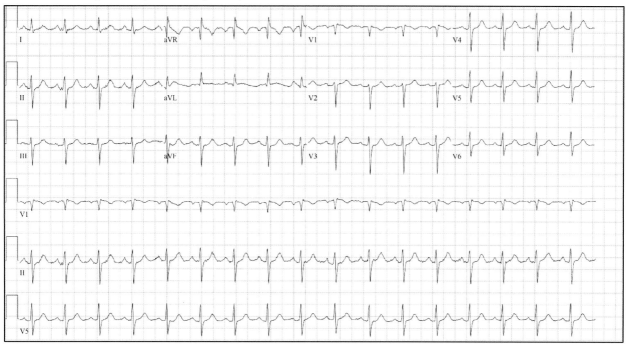

Left anterior fascicular block

Rate: 103 Rhythm: sinus tachycardia Axis: left axis deviation Intervals: normal
Ischemia: none

What are the five causes of left axis deviation?
1) Left ventricular hypertrophy
2) Left bundle branch block/paced rhythm/ventricular ectopy
3) Left anterior fascicular block (LAFB),
4) Pre-excitation
5) Inferior myocardial infarction (inferior Q waves)

What part of the conduction system is affected?
The left anterior fascicle is blocked. Criteria for diagnosing LAFB includes: left axis deviation (usually > 45 deg); small q waves with large R waves ("qR complexes") in I and aVL; small r waves with large S waves ("rS complexes") in II, III, and aVF; normal or slightly prolonged QRS duration (80-110 ms).[8] If there is a leftward shift in the axis greater than 45 degrees, it is almost certainly the result of a LAFB because no other condition generates such extreme left shift.

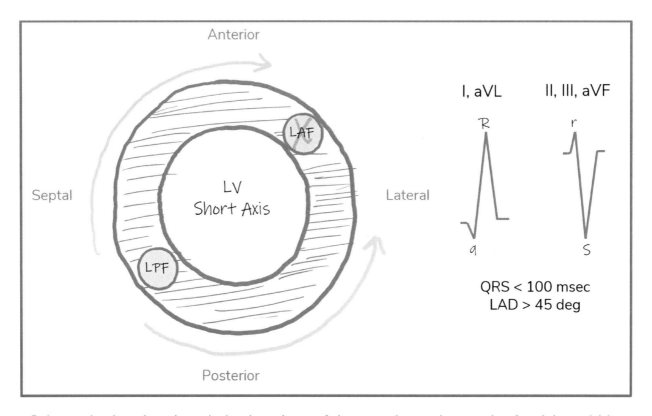

Schematic showing the relative locations of the anterior and posterior fascicles within the left ventricle. The curved blue arrows demonstrate the direction of depolarization from the posterobasal segment of the left ventricle to the anterolateral segment (given the blocked left anterior fascicle). LV, left ventricle; LPF, left posterior fascicle; LAF, left anterior fascicle; LAD, left axis deviation.

What is the significance of this finding?

In isolation, LAFB is not clinically significant. When seen in combination with other conduction system disease (i.e. a right bundle branch block and first-degree atrioventricular block) in the setting of syncope, it may signal intermittent complete heart block. The diseased area of the conduction system is the left anterior fascicle of the interventricular conduction system.

#6 – 62 yo F p/w dyspnea

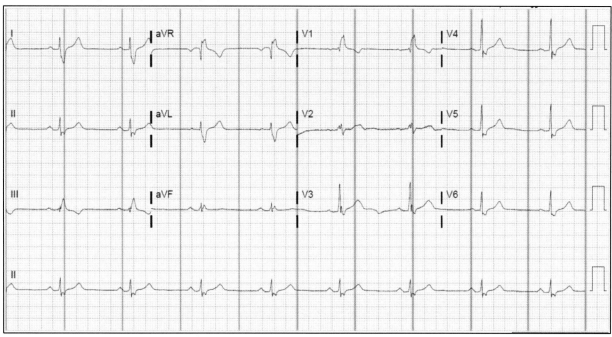

Rate: _____ Rhythm: _____ Axis: _____ Intervals: _____ Ischemia: _____

What are the causes of bifascicular block?

What is a "tri"fascicular block and why is it a misnomer?

#6 – 62 yo F p/w dyspnea

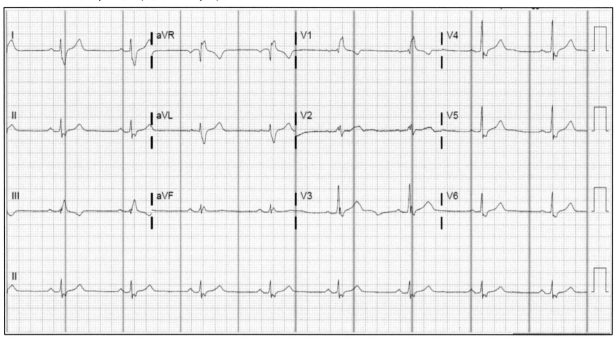

Bifascicular block (RBBB, LPFB)

<u>Rate</u>: 48 <u>Rhythm</u>: sinus bradycardia <u>Axis</u>: right axis deviation <u>Intervals</u>: wide QRS
<u>Ischemia</u>: none

What are the causes of bifascicular block?

When two fascicles are blocked, it is termed bifascicular block. Causes include ischemic heart disease (40-60% cases), hypertension (20-25%), aortic stenosis, anterior myocardial infarction (occurs acutely in 5-7%), primary degenerative disease of the conducting system (Lenegre's/Lev's disease), congenital heart disease, and hyperkalemia.[8] Recall that right bundle branch block (RBBB) is not normally associated with axis deviation (unlike left bundle branch block). The right axis deviation is explained by the presence of a left posterior fascicular block (LPFB).

What is a "tri"fascicular block and why is it a misnomer?

Trifascicular block is a term used to describe a bifascicular block with first or second-degree atrioventricular (AV) block. In the setting of pre-existing conduction disease (i.e. bifascicular block), the first or second-degree AV block likely represents a delay of conduction through the remaining conducting fascicle (Hisian delay). Since conduction through the remaining fascicle is delayed and not blocked, the term is a misnomer.[19] Myocardial infarctions associated with pre-existing conduction disease have significantly worse prognoses.[20,21]

#7 – 72 yo F p/w anxiety

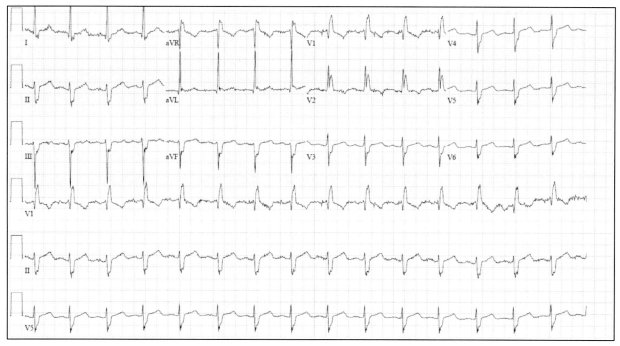

Rate: _____　Rhythm: _____　Axis: _____　Intervals: _____　Ischemia: _____

When are fascicular blocks clinically relevant?

#7 – 72 yo F p/w anxiety

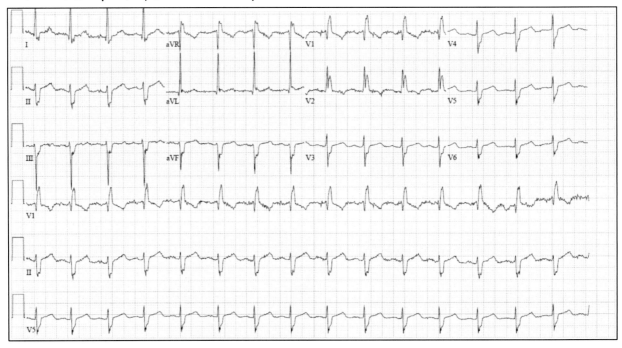

Bifascicular block (RBBB, LAFB)

Rate: 90 Rhythm: sinus Axis: left axis deviation Intervals: wide QRS Ischemia: none

When are fascicular blocks clinically relevant?

When isolated, fascicular blocks are generally clinically insignificant but warrant additional considerations when associated with additional conduction disturbances (i.e. bi or trifascicular block).[4] The term "trifascicular block" refers to conduction disease of all three fascicles – the right bundle branch, the left posterior and left anterior fascicles.[5] It is usually characterized electrocardiographically by a bifascicular block and a delay in conduction through the remaining fascicle, represented by a prolonged PR interval. Patients with bi or trifascicular block are at increased risk for deterioration to complete heart block. In the setting of symptoms concerning for bradycardia (e.g. syncope, presyncope, hemodynamic instability), permanent pacing is potentially indicated.

#8 – 60 yo M p/w dyspnea on exertion

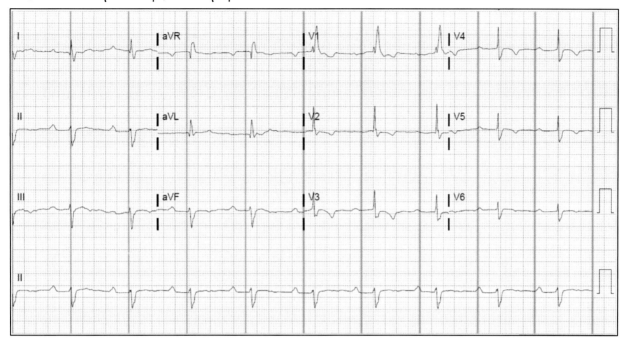

Rate: _____ Rhythm: _____ Axis: _____ Intervals: _____ Ischemia: _____

Is this patient a candidate for a pacemaker?

#8 – 60 yo M p/w dyspnea on exertion

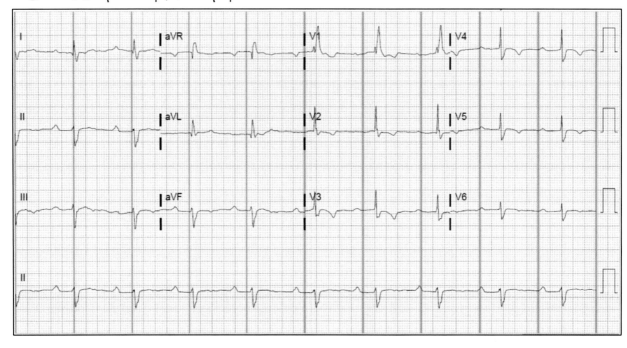

Trifascicular disease

Rate: 60 Rhythm: sinus Axis: left axis deviation Intervals: wide QRS Ischemia: lateral T wave inversions

Is this patient a candidate for a pacemaker?

This patient has trifascicular disease as evidenced by the right bundle branch block, left anterior fascicular block, and first-degree atrioventricular block. As mentioned in case #6 of this unit, first-degree atrioventricular block in this setting likely represents delayed conduction through the remaining, yet diseased, left posterior fascicle. This patient needs to see a cardiologist and, at minimum, needs ambulatory electrocardiographic monitoring to evaluate for intermittent complete heart block, potentially necessitating pacemaker placement.[8]

Unit 3

Alternative Explanations for ST Elevation
Right Heart Strain
Global Subendocardial Ischemia
Left Ventricular Hypertrophy
Narrow Complex Tachycardia

#1 – 21 yo p/w altered mental status after vehicle accident

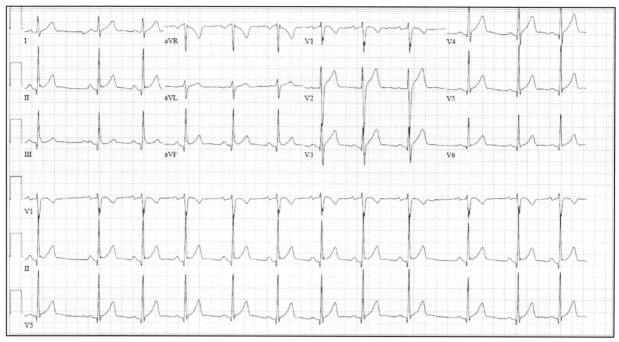

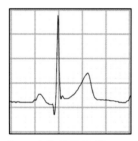

Lead II QRS Complex

What phenomenon explains the ST elevations in this ECG?

What are the features of this condition?

What is the clinical significance of this phenomenon?

#1 – 21 yo p/w altered mental status after vehicle accident

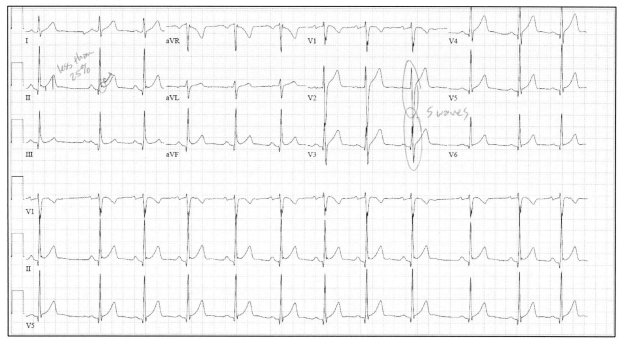

handwritten annotations: "less than 25%", "S waves"

Early repolarization or the J wave pattern

Rate: 96 Rhythm: sinus Axis: normal Intervals: normal Ischemia: Diffuse ST elevation without reciprocal changes

What phenomenon explains the ST elevations in this ECG?

(Benign) early repolarization (BER) or the J wave pattern. *Good! STEMI mimicker*

What are the features of this condition?

Features include diffuse ST elevations that are most pronounced in the precordial leads (typically V2-5) and in proportion to the amplitude of the QRS complex. The degree of ST elevation in V6 should be less than 25% the height of the QRS.[22] J point notching (i.e. "fishhook") can be seen. The T waves should be concordant (same direction as QRS), and there should not be any reciprocal changes.[2]

When you see ST elevations, ask yourself: 1) are there reciprocal changes? 2) is there tombstone morphology? STEMI needs to have a ST:T wave amplitude change > 25% of QRS

51

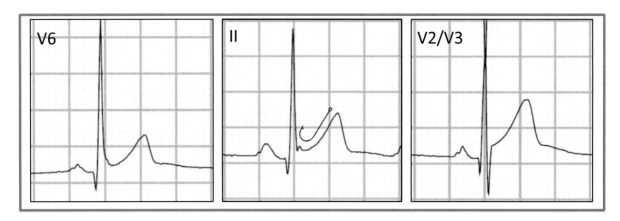

ST elevation can be clearly seen in the above leads. Lead II has J point notching (i.e. "fishhook"), characteristic of early repolarization.

What is the clinical significance of this phenomenon?

BER has traditionally been considered benign, but newer data suggests that the prevalence of the J wave pattern is higher among patients with idiopathic ventricular fibrillation. It is unclear, however, whether this finding has any significance among asymptomatic individuals.[23]

#2 – 67 yo M c̄ h/o STEMI p/w chest pain

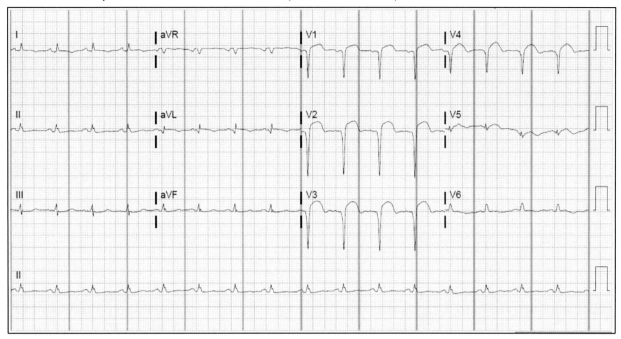

Rate: _____ Rhythm: _____ Axis: _____ Intervals: _____ Ischemia: _____

What finding would you expected on bedside echocardiography?

What ECG features suggest this diagnosis?

#2 – 67 yo M c̄ h/o STEMI p/w chest pain

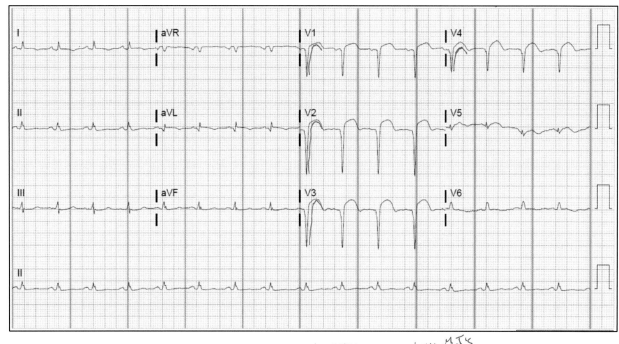

Left ventricular aneurysm *commonly seen in large, untreated anterior MI's*

<u>Rate</u>: 96　<u>Rhythm</u>: sinus　<u>Axis</u>: normal　<u>Intervals</u>: normal　<u>Ischemia</u>: large Q waves and ST elevations in V1-V4

What finding would you expected on bedside echocardiography?

Findings of left ventricular aneurysm on bedside echocardiography include ballooning at the apex of the left ventricle or apical akinesias.[24]

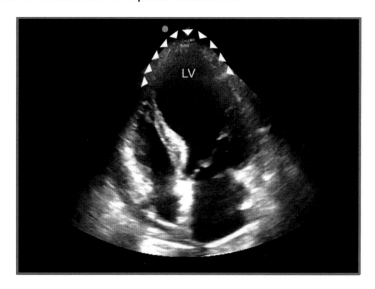

Apical four chamber echocardiogram showing severe balloon-like dilation of the left ventricle (LV) apex (triangles).

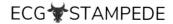

What ECG features suggest this diagnosis?

The usual ECG findings of left ventricular aneurysm include ST elevation that persists more than two weeks after STEMI, deep Q waves, and the absence of reciprocal ST depressions.[25] Based on the concept of "proportionality" (the idea that the T-wave amplitude has an expected proportion to the QRS amplitude), two rules to differentiate anterior ST-elevation myocardial infarction from left ventricular aneurysm were validated for patients with suspected acute coronary syndrome and troponin I level less than 5 ng/dL. Note that neither rule's test characteristics are sufficient enough to rule out ST-elevation myocardial infarction in the symptomatic patient.

Rule 1

$$\frac{sum\ of\ T\ wave\ amplitudes\ V1 + V2 + V3 + V4}{sum\ of\ QRS\ amplitudes\ V1 + V2 + V3 + V4} > 0.22$$

Rule 2

$$\frac{T\ wave\ amplitude}{QRS\ amplitude}\ In\ any\ lead\ V1, V2, V3,\ or\ V4\ \geq 0.36$$

Rule 1 ~87% accuracy, Rule 2 ~89% accuracy[26]

In the age of reperfusion, left ventricular aneurysms have become quite rare, but in the absence of reperfusion, it is a common structural complication of acute myocardial infarction, occurring in 35% to 64% of anterior myocardial infarctions.[27,28]

#3 – 80 yo F p/w typical chest pain

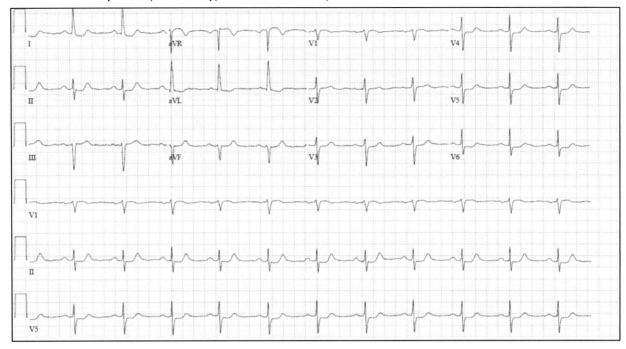

Rate: _____ Rhythm: _____ Axis: _____ Intervals: _____ Ischemia: _____

What type of coronary disease is this ECG pattern associated with?

What are alternative explanations for this pattern?

- worse w/ exertion
- radiation (extremities)
- diaphoresis
- vomiting   *2/4 signs or symptoms*

#3 – 80 yo F p/w typical chest pain

- I don't see diffuse ST dep...
- when is something diffuse? when multiple, all leads

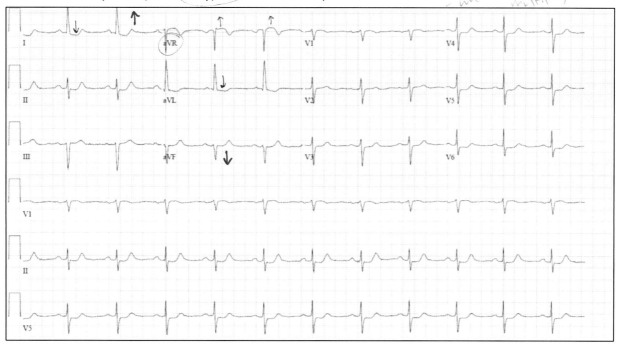

Multivessel disease

Rate: 66 Rhythm: sinus Axis: left axis deviation Intervals: normal Ischemia: diffuse ST depression with 1 mm ST elevation in aVR

What type of coronary disease is this ECG pattern associated with?

Multilead ST depression with ST elevation in aVR (≥1 mm) is a strong predictor of left main or triple vessel disease.[29] In the setting of acute coronary syndrome, the European Society of Cardiology guidelines recommend this pattern as an indication for emergent reperfusion.[12] It is important, however, to recognize that the clinical context should support this diagnosis (i.e. history is consistent with acute coronary syndrome), and not one of the other many diagnoses that can cause this pattern. This patient had a history consistent with acute coronary syndrome and had a coronary bypass the following day.

What are alternative explanations for this pattern?

There are many explanations for this pattern including left ventricular hypertrophy, hypokalemia, pulmonary embolism, and any condition that creates a supply/demand mismatch like acute blood loss, sepsis, respiratory failure, tachydysrhythmias, or aortic stenosis.[30,31]

#4 – 63 yo F p/w dyspnea

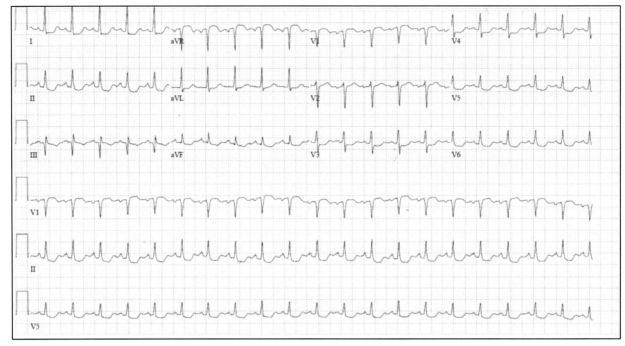

Rate: _____ Rhythm: _____ Axis: _____ Intervals: _____ Ischemia: _____

How might the differential diagnosis for multilead ST depressions with coexistent aVR ST elevation change for this patient's presenting complaint?

#4 – 63 yo F p/w dyspnea

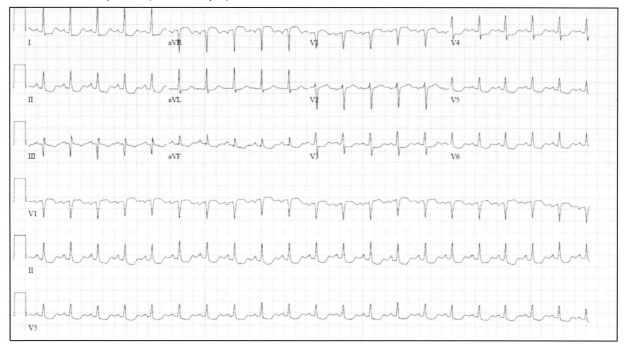

Pulmonary embolism

Rate: 126 Rhythm: sinus tachycardia Axis: normal Intervals: normal Ischemia: diffuse ST depression with > 1 mm ST elevation in aVR

How might the differential diagnosis for multilead ST depressions with coexistent aVR ST elevation change for this patient's presenting complaint?

While this pattern has been recognized as a strong predictor of left main coronary artery or 3-vessel disease, occlusive coronary artery disease is not the only cause of this ECG pattern. Frequently, this pattern results from nonocclusive causes such as baseline left ventricular hypertrophy or conditions that create a supply-demand mismatch such as acute blood loss, sepsis, respiratory failure, tachydysrhythmias, and aortic stenosis.[32] In one series of 133 patients showing this ECG pattern, only 28% had acute coronary syndromes, whereas 45% had hypertensive heart disease.[30] Although the mechanism is not clear, it is postulated that acute pulmonary embolism can lead to profound right and left ventricular ischemia, causing aVR-STE, which can lead to a misdiagnosis of primary ischemic disease.[33] This patient had a massive pulmonary embolism and was hemodynamically unstable. Thrombolytics were given and two hours later the ischemic ECG findings resolved.[31]

#5 – 76 yo M p/w syncope

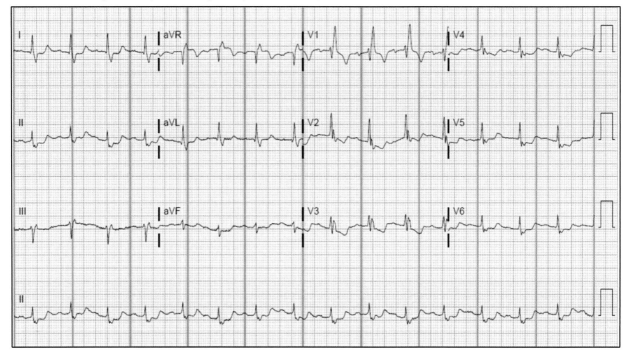

Rate: _____ Rhythm: _____ Axis: _____ Intervals: _____ Ischemia: _____

How might the differential diagnosis for multilead ST depressions with coexistent aVR ST elevation change for this patient's presenting complaint?

#5 – 76 yo M p/w syncope

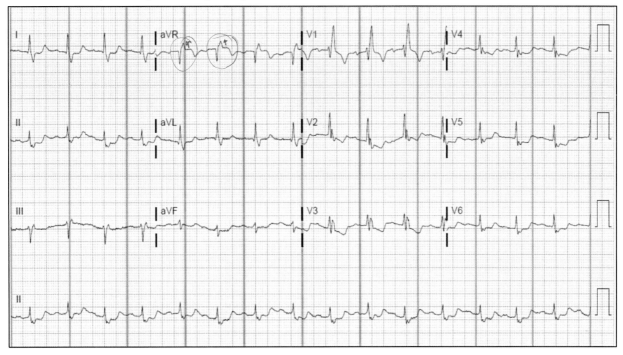

Global subendocardial ischemia

<u>Rate</u>: 90 <u>Rhythm</u>: sinus <u>Axis</u>: normal <u>Intervals</u>: wide QRS, prolonged PR <u>Ischemia</u>: diffuse ST depressions with ST elevation in aVR (>1 mm)

How might the differential diagnosis for multilead ST depressions with coexistent aVR ST elevation change for this patient's presenting complaint?

This patient suffered from acute anemia due to upper gastrointestinal bleeding. The ischemic findings resolved after adequate transfusion. This case serves as a reminder to keep a broad differential diagnosis when the pattern of global subendocardial ischemia (multilead ST depression and coexistent aVR ST elevation) is encountered. Of note, this patient also has a right bundle branch block and a first-degree atrioventricular block.

#6 – 51 yo F p/w atypical chest pain

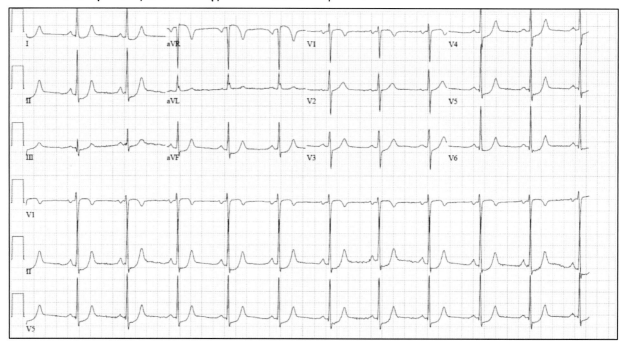

Rate: _____ Rhythm: _____ Axis: _____ Intervals: _____ Ischemia: _____

How might the differential diagnosis for multilead ST depressions with coexistent aVR ST elevation change for this patient's presenting complaint?

#6 – 51 yo F p/w atypical chest pain

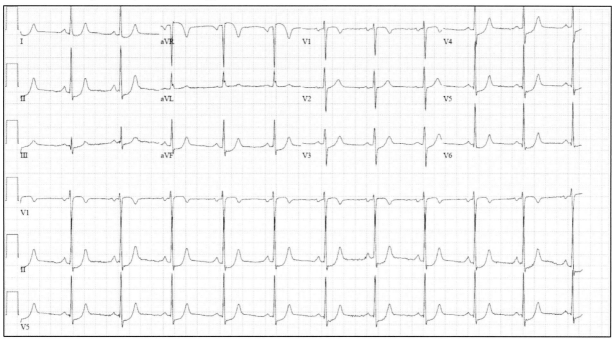

Myocarditis

Rate: 66 Rhythm: sinus Axis: normal Intervals: normal Ischemia: diffuse ST depression with > 1 mm ST elevation in aVR

How might the differential diagnosis for multilead ST depressions with coexistent aVR ST elevation change for this patient's presenting complaint?
This is yet another case that serves as a reminder to keep a broad differential diagnosis when the pattern of global subendocardial ischemia (multilead ST depression and coexistent aVR ST elevation) is encountered. This patient was ultimately diagnosed with myocarditis and hypokalemia, both of which can cause this pattern.

This pt was cath lab but had a clean cath – just a reminder to keep broad differential

#7 – 69 yo M p/w dyspnea & chest pain

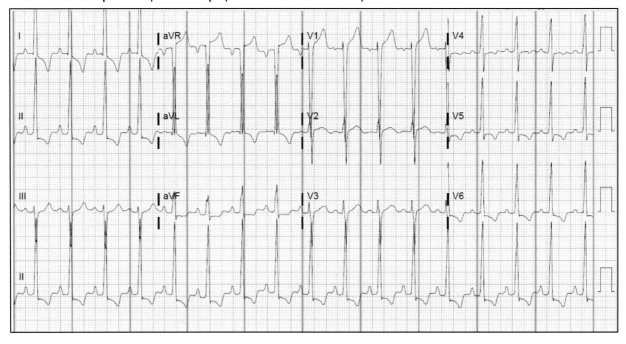

Rate: _____ Rhythm: _____ Axis: _____ Intervals: _____ Ischemia: _____

What are the electrocardiographic criteria used to diagnose left ventricular hypertrophy?

#7 – 69 yo M p/w dyspnea & chest pain

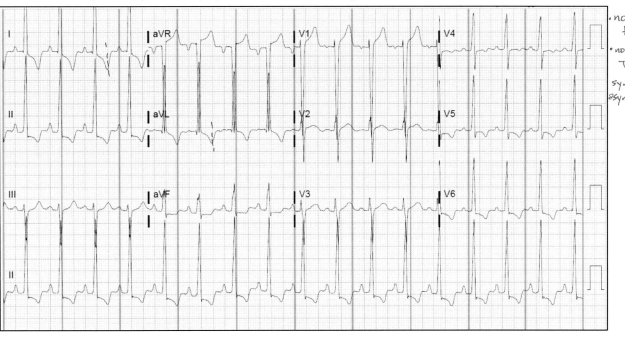

Handwritten margin notes:
- note: high voltage throughout EKG
- note: asymmetric T wave depression symmetry usually ST asymmetric usually strain

Left ventricular hypertrophy

<u>Rate</u>: 100 <u>Rhythm</u>: sinus tachycardia <u>Axis</u>: normal <u>Intervals</u>: slightly widened QRS

<u>Ischemia</u>: diffuse ST depression with > 1 mm ST elevation in aVR and asymmetric T wave inversions in the inferolateral leads

What are the electrocardiographic criteria used to diagnose left ventricular hypertrophy?

There are several criteria out there for left ventricular hypertrophy, and none of them are particularly sensitive. They're all less than 50% sensitive, but they're usually quite specific - 85 to 90%. The most cited criteria are the Sokolow-Lyon and the Cornell criteria, which consider voltage amplitude. There are also ST/T wave changes associated with LVH that may increase the specificity when seen. Namely, lateral ST depressions and asymmetric T wave inversions like the ones seen in this ECG.[34]

Select Electrocardiographic Criteria for Left Ventricular Hypertrophy	
Sokolow-Lyon Criteria	S V_1 + R $V_{5,6}$ > 35 mm OR R aVL > 11 mm
Cornell Criteria	R aVL + S V_3 > 28 mm for men OR > 20 mm for women

In one series of 133 patients with multilead ST depression and aVR ST elevation, 45% were the result of the changes produced by left ventricular hypertrophy (LVH).[30]

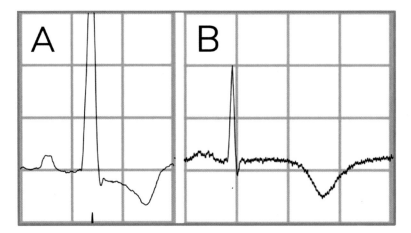

Panel A is a complex from V6 of this case demonstrating a QRS tall complex (extending 6 mm beyond the margin of the image) and an asymmetric T wave inversion characteristic of the "strain" pattern of left ventricular hypertrophy. The "strain" morphology in Panel A is contrasted with the symmetric T wave inversion in Panel B, consistent with ischemia. Panel B shows a complex from V6 in a patient found to have a critical stenosis of the left anterior descending artery. The patient in Panel A had a heart catheterization which demonstrated patent coronary vessels.

#8 – 44 yo F p/w chest pain

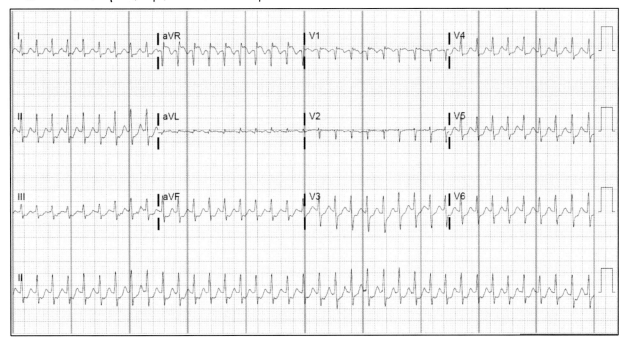

Rate: _____ Rhythm: _____ Axis: _____ Intervals: _____ Ischemia: _____

What is the differential for regular, narrow complex tachycardia?

#8 – 44 yo F p/w chest pain

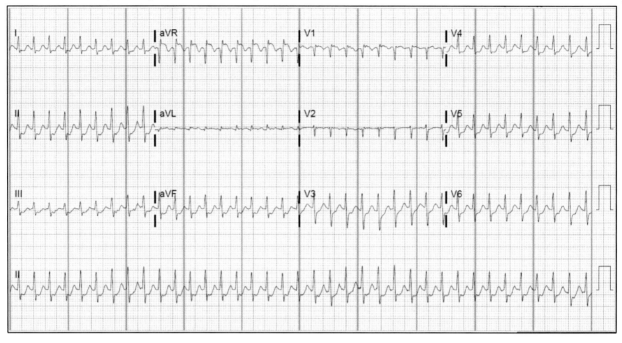

Supraventricular tachycardia

Rate: 220   Rhythm: supraventricular tachycardia   Axis: normal   Intervals: normal
Ischemia: diffuse ST depression with > 1 mm ST elevation in aVR

What is the differential for regular, narrow complex tachycardia?

The differential includes sinus tachycardia, atrioventricular nodal reentrant tachycardia (AVNRT), atrial flutter with fixed conduction, atrial tachycardia, and atrioventricular reentrant tachycardia. Rates at this speed strongly suggest atrioventricular nodal reentrant tachycardia.[35] The term supraventricular tachycardia technically refers to any tachycardic arrythmia arising from a focus above the ventricles (i.e. atria or atrioventricular node), but practically it is often used synonymously with AVNRT. AVNRT refers to a reentrant tachycardia within the atrioventricular node that results from a dual pathway (one fast, one slow), found in 10 to 35% of normal people.[2,36]

The aVR ST elevation pattern is expected with supraventricular tachycardia and this pattern has no significance in this setting. Rate-related waveform compression causes exaggerated ST changes, so it is important to not over diagnosis ischemia until the rate is addressed.

#9 – 62 yo M p/w chest pain

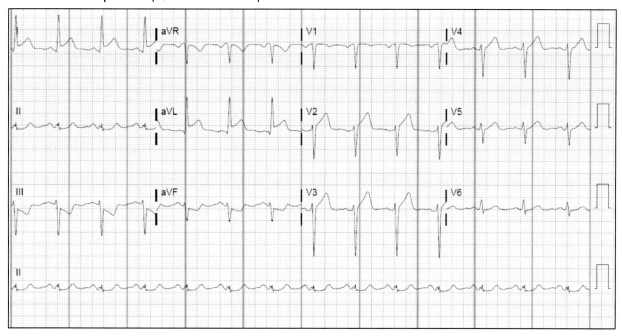

Rate: _____ Rhythm: _____ Axis: _____ Intervals: _____ Ischemia: _____

What is the anatomic distribution of the ST changes?

What artery is most commonly involved?

#9 – 62 yo M p/w chest pain

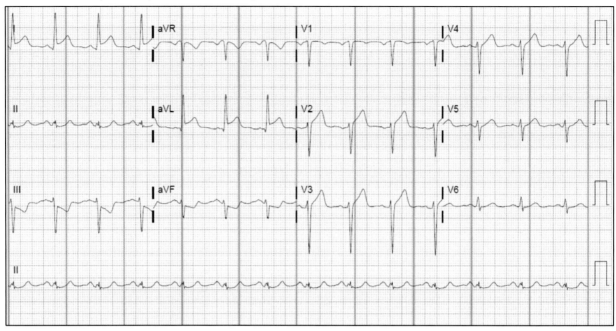

High lateral STEMI

due to ischemia

Rate: 84 Rhythm: sinus Axis: left axis deviation Intervals: normal Ischemia: ST elevation in I and aVL with reciprocal ST depression in II, III, and aVF

What is the anatomic distribution of the ST changes?

This is a high lateral STEMI (I and aVL). There is some ST elevation in V2 but not technically enough to call STEMI per the formal criteria. Beware of this level of ST measurement precision as you may likely miss the forest for the trees.

ST-elevation Myocardial Infarction as defined in the 4th Universal Definition of Myocardial Infarction[37]
New ST-elevation at the J-point in two contiguous leads with the cut-point ≥1 mm in all leads other than leads V2-V3 where the following cut-points apply: • ≥2 mm in men ≥40 years • ≥2.5 mm in men < 40 years, or • ≥1.5 mm in women regardless of age

International definition of ST-elevation myocardial infarction.

What artery is most commonly involved?

The first diagonal branch (D1) of the left anterior descending artery, sometimes left circumflex.[38]

Unit 4

Alternative Explanations for ST Elevation
Electrolyte Disturbances
Myocardial Infarction and Conduction Disturbances
Early Signs of Ischemia

#1 – 37 yo F p/w sharp pleuritic chest pain

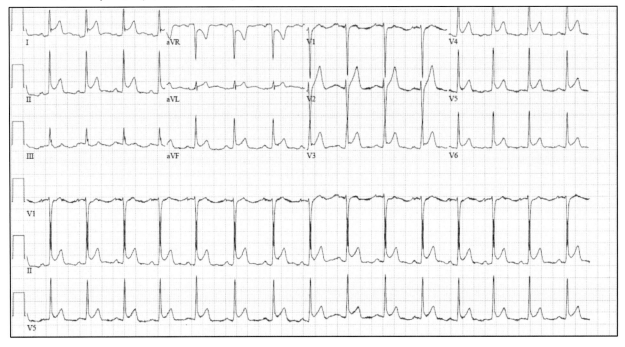

Rate: _____ Rhythm: _____ Axis: _____ Intervals: _____ Ischemia: _____

What is the diagnosis and how is it made?

What is the natural ECG progression of this disease process?

What are the treatment options?

differs from video

#1 – 3̶7̶ ⁱ⁷ yo F̶ ᴹ p/w sharp pleuritic chest pain

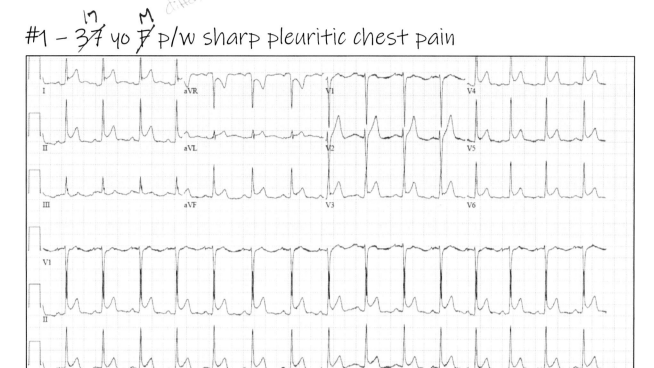

Acute pericarditis

Rate: 60 Rhythm: sinus Axis: normal Intervals: normal Ischemia: diffuse ST elevations without reciprocal changes

What is the diagnosis and how is it made?

Acute pericarditis. The diagnosis is made by meeting 2 of 4 criteria[2,39]:

1) Typical symptoms (pleuritic sharp chest pain better when leaning forward)
2) New pericardial effusion
3) Presence of friction rub
4) Typical ECG findings

Differentiating pericarditis from STEMI can be challenging, but features that suggest pericarditis over STEMI include any of the following: diffuse concave up ST elevations without reciprocal changes, PR depression, PR elevation in aVR, ST-elevation in lead II greater than lead III, and Spodick's sign – down-sloping of the TP segment.[40] It is important to note that the test characteristics of any single electrocardiographic feature is insufficient to rule in/out pericarditis, and that the feature with the highest odds ratio for predicting STEMI is reciprocal ST-depressions.[40]

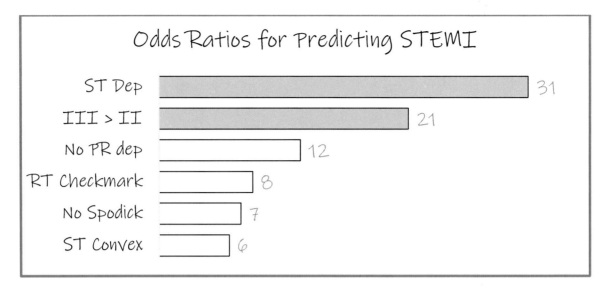

Odds ratios of various ECG findings for predicting STEMI vs. pericarditis. Reciprocal ST depressions (ST dep) and ST-elevation in III>II are the strongest predictors of STEMI.[40]

What is the natural ECG progression of this disease process?

The first two weeks are characterized by the above findings. Over several weeks, the ST elevation resolves, and the T waves flatten. Next the T waves invert. Finally, over several weeks the ECG returns to the patient's baseline.[41]

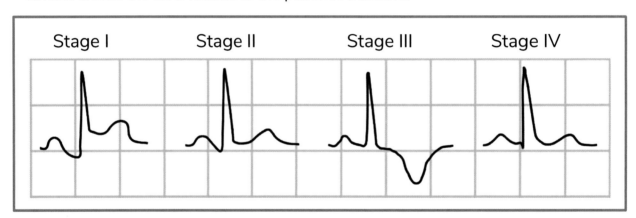

Morphologic features of the various stages of pericarditis.

What are the treatment options?

Colchicine for 3 months and NSAIDs/aspirin tapered over 3-4 weeks are first line in patients without contraindications.[42] It's reasonable to prescribe a proton pump inhibitor also. Corticosteroids are reserved for patients with colchicine/NSAID/aspirin contraindication and are not preferred as they are associated with increased recurrence.[39]

#2 – 69 yo M p/w altered mental status

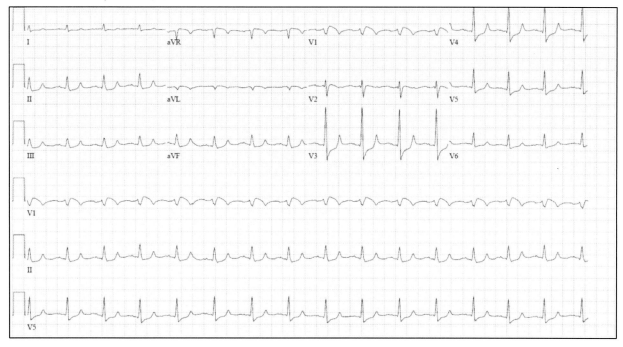

Rate: _____ Rhythm: _____ Axis: _____ Intervals: _____ Ischemia: _____

What treatment options in the ED do you have for this patient and how do they work?

With this condition, what three ECG features predict adverse outcomes?

#2 – 69 yo M p/w altered mental status

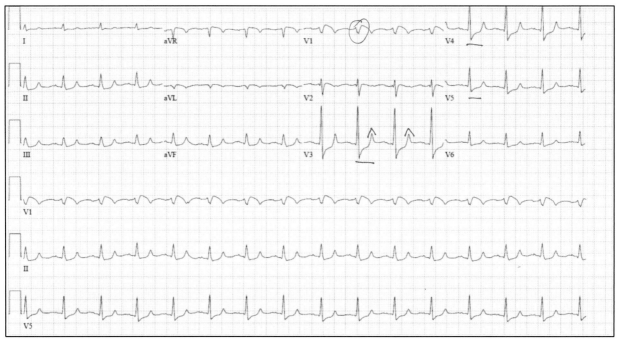

Hyperkalemia-induced ST changes

<u>Rate</u>: 96   <u>Rhythm</u>: sinus   <u>Axis</u>: normal   <u>Intervals</u>: wide QRS   <u>Ischemia</u>: ST elevation in V1, inferolateral ST depressions, peaked T waves

What treatment options in the ED do you have for this patient and how do they work?

This patient was hyperkalemic and found to be in diabetic ketoacidosis. He was given intravenous calcium with resolution of the ECG changes (see next page). Membrane stabilizers include calcium and hypertonic saline. Intracellular potassium shifters include insulin/glucose, beta-agonists, and sodium bicarbonate in acidotic patients. *watch out for this* Potassium eliminators include loop diuretics and kayexalate. Newer medications to promote gastrointestinal excretion hold promise (patiromer and sodium zirconium cyclosilicate).[43]

With this condition, what three ECG features predict adverse outcomes?

1) Bradycardia < 50 bpm   *slow*
2) QRS > 110 ms   *wide*
3) Junctional rhythm

Notice that peaked T waves were not found to predict acute adverse outcomes.[44]

ECG🐂STAMPEDE

#2 – 69 yo M p/w altered mental status (after calcium)

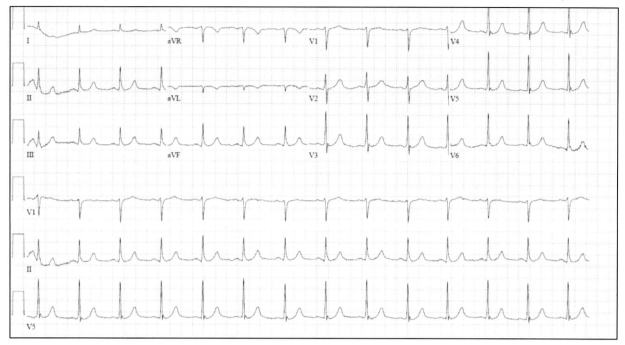

Hyperacute T waves   look at proportion to QRS

vs

Peaked T waves

#3 – 31 yo M p/w weakness

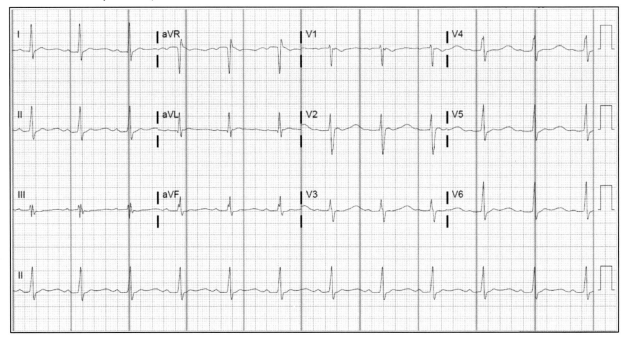

Rate: _____ Rhythm: _____ Axis: _____ Intervals: _____ Ischemia: _____

What electrolyte disturbances cause the interval problem seen in this ECG?

#3 – 31 yo M p/w weakness

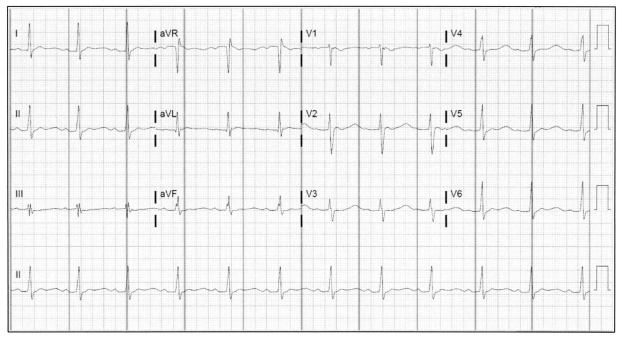

Hypokalemia

<u>Rate</u>: 72 <u>Rhythm</u>: sinus <u>Axis</u>: normal <u>Intervals</u>: prolonged QT interval <u>Ischemia</u>: none

What electrolyte disturbances cause the interval problem seen in this ECG?

Hypokalemia, hypomagnesemia, and hypocalcemia can all cause a prolongation of the QT interval. While hypokalemia and hypomagnesemia both delay the repolarization phase (phase 3) of the of the cardiac action potential (creating wide-based T waves, U waves, or a fusion of both), hypocalcemia prolongs the QT interval by way of extending the plateau phase (phase 2) of the cardiac action potential (lengthening the ST segment but with a normal T wave). This ECG is consistent with hypokalemia and/or hypomagnesemia.[45]

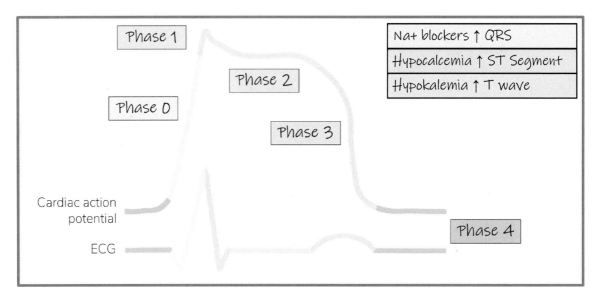

This schematic demonstrates the various phases of the cardiac action potential as they relate to the ECG waveform. In phase 0, fast acting voltage-gated sodium channels open and a rapid influx of sodium results. Sodium channel blocking agents tend to predominantly affect phase 0 and widen the QRS complex. During phase 2, voltage-gated potassium (efflux) and calcium (influx) channels tend to maintain a relative potential plateau. Since phase 2 represents the ST segment, hypocalcemia tends to produce a long ST segment, but a normal T wave. Finally, in phase 3, potassium channels allow more potassium to leak and "repolarize" the cell. Hypokalemia tends to delay this phase, creating broad-based T waves, U waves, and T-U fusions.

#4 – 49 yo M p/w chest pain

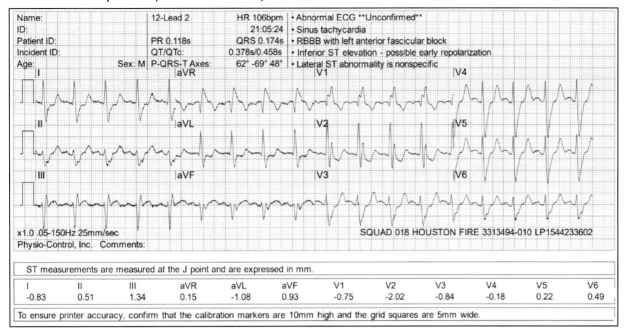

Rate: _____ Rhythm: _____ Axis: _____ Intervals: _____ Ischemia: _____

What conduction disturbances are present?

What are the subtle ischemic findings?

#4 - 49 yo M p/w chest pain

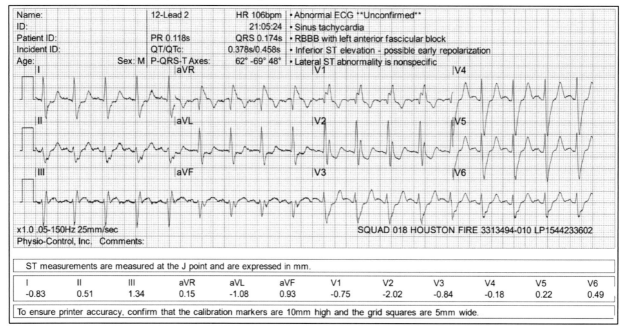

I	II	III	aVR	aVL	aVF	V1	V2	V3	V4	V5	V6
-0.83	0.51	1.34	0.15	-1.08	0.93	-0.75	-2.02	-0.84	-0.18	0.22	0.49

Subtle inferior STEMI and bifascicular block

Rate: 106 Rhythm: sinus Axis: left axis deviation Intervals: wide QRS Ischemia: inferior ST segment straightening with reciprocal ST depression in aVL

What conduction disturbances are present?

The ECG shows a bifascicular block (right bundle branch block and left anterior fascicular block).

What are the subtle ischemic findings?

There are straightened inferior ST segments and reciprocal ST depressions in aVL. ST straightening refers to morphologic changes of the ST segment that can be an early ischemic finding. Some consider a bifascicular block with typical chest pain to be an indication for emergent reperfusion. In fact, the latest European guidelines suggest emergent reperfusion for patients with acute coronary syndrome and a new right bundle branch block.[12] So-called "typical" features of chest pain include exertional symptoms, associated nausea with vomiting or diaphoresis, and pain radiation.[46,47] The infarct-related changes on this ECG continued to evolve and are more evident on the subsequent ECG (next page).

#4 – 49 yo M p/w chest pain (15 min after initial ECG)

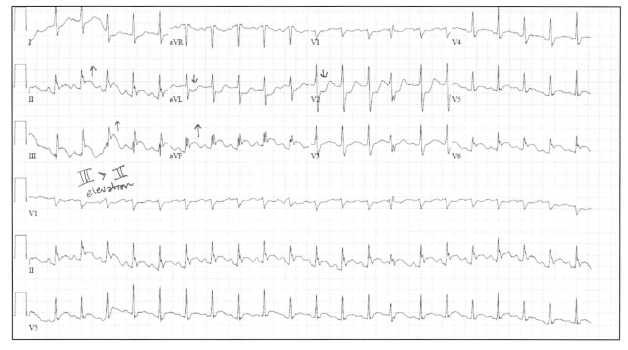

Inferior STEMI

Rate: 126 Rhythm: sinus Axis: left axis deviation Intervals: normal Ischemia: inferolateral STEMI with reciprocal ST depression in V2 and aVL

About one third of inferior infarcts are associated with right ventricular infarcts (caused by right coronary artery occlusion proximal to the right ventricular branch, as with this case). These are important to recognize because patients with right ventricular infarcts have more complications and poorer short-term prognoses. Complications include hypotension (that will respond to fluids), bradycardia, and atrioventricular block. Avoidance of preload reducers like nitrites is recommended. It is important to recognize the findings of right ventricular infarct which include inferior wall ST elevation with the greatest magnitude ST elevation in lead III, ST elevation in V1, and ST elevation in right-sided precordial leads (specifically V4R).[3,48] Right-sided precordial leads can be obtained by reversing the precordial leads across the right chest wall. Curiously, the right bundle branch bock disappeared on this repeat ECG.

#5 – 12 yo F p/w dyspnea, arrested on arrival

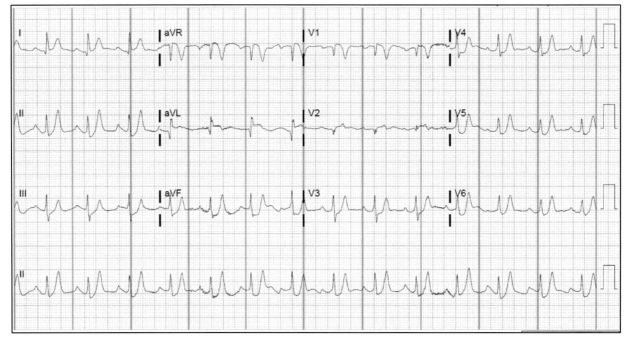

Rate: _____ Rhythm: _____ Axis: _____ Intervals: _____ Ischemia: _____

What are deWinter T waves and what do they indicate?

What diagnosis is suggested by the lack of a clear anatomic distribution of the ischemic changes in this ECG?

#5 – 12 yo F p/w dyspnea, arrested on arrival

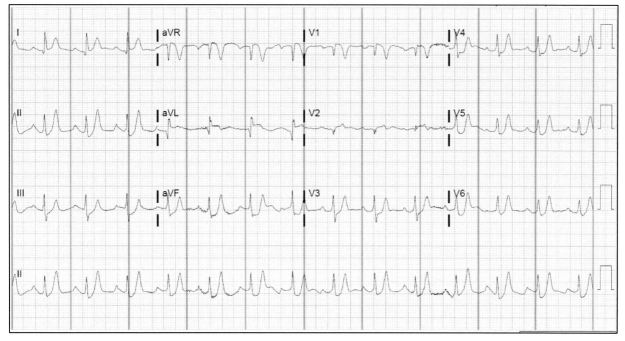

Hyperacute T waves

Rate: 84　Rhythm: sinus　Axis: normal　Intervals: normal　Ischemia: diffuse upsloping
ST depressions with hyperacute T waves, ST elevations in I and aVL

What are deWinter T waves and what do they indicate?

In 2008, deWinter described a pattern of ST depressions and hyperacute, or "rocket"
T waves in the precordial leads that indicated proximal left anterior descending
occlusion. The pattern was initially described as static but has since been described
as dynamic, too. It is believed to occur in about 2% of anterior myocardial
infarctions.[49,50] deWinter T waves have been described in myocarditis where the
phenomenon is consistent with general myocardial injury rather than coronary
occlusion.

means huge ischemia that needs to be intervened on

What diagnosis is suggested by the lack of a clear anatomic distribution of the ischemic changes in this ECG?

This patient's troponin came back > 30 ng/mL and she was transferred for
extracorporeal membrane oxygenation. She was diagnosed with myocarditis.

Unit 5

Causes of Sudden Cardiac Death
Right Heart Strain
Prolonged QT
Environmental Emergencies
Repolarization Abnormalities

#1 – 28 yo M p/w syncope

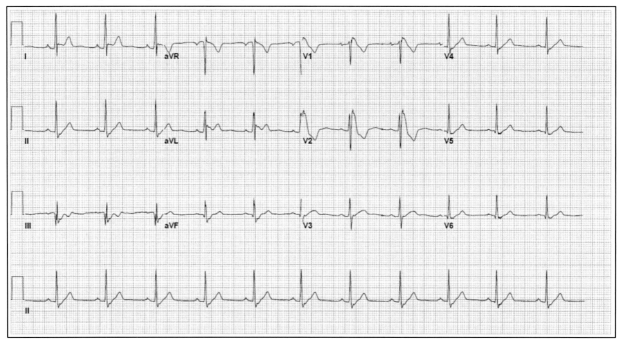

Rate: _____ Rhythm: _____ Axis: _____ Intervals: _____ Ischemia: _____

What's the diagnosis?

What's the disposition and management?

What conditions can expose/unmask the diagnosis?

#1 – 28 yo M p/w syncope

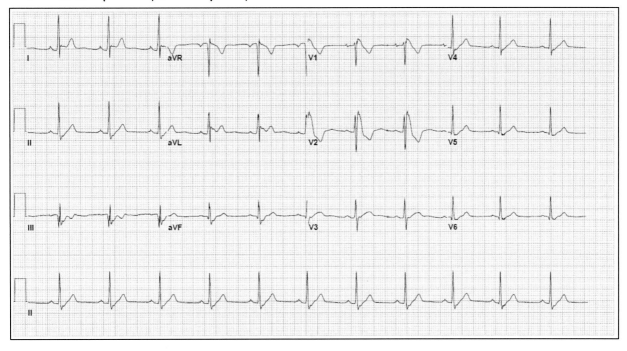

Brugada pattern type I, coved-type

Rate: 66 Rhythm: sinus Axis: normal Intervals: normal Ischemia: RSR' pattern in V1/V2 with down-sloping ST elevations and T wave inversions

What's the diagnosis?

Type I, or coved-type Brugada pattern. Brugada syndrome is a sodium channelopathy with a characteristic ECG pattern (ST segment elevation of ≥2 mm with a coved-type morphology in ≥1 right precordial lead) and an increased risk of sudden cardiac death, in the absence of gross structural heart disease.[51]

What's the disposition and management?

This patient should be presumed to have had a ventricular dysrhythmia and should be admitted for an automatic implantable internal cardioverter-defibrillator.

What conditions can expose/unmask the diagnosis?

Patients with Brugada syndrome may only manifest typical Brugada morphologies when the channelopathy is unmasked by infections, ischemia, drug use (such as ajmaline, flecainide, or procainamide), or hypokalemia.[51] Drugs known to unmask the pattern can be found at www.brugadadrugs.org.

#2 – 33 yo M p/w dizziness

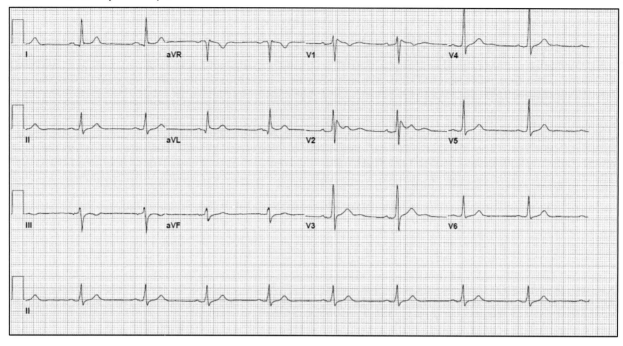

Rate: _____ Rhythm: _____ Axis: _____ Intervals: _____ Ischemia: _____

What's the disposition and management?

#2 – 33 yo M p/w dizziness

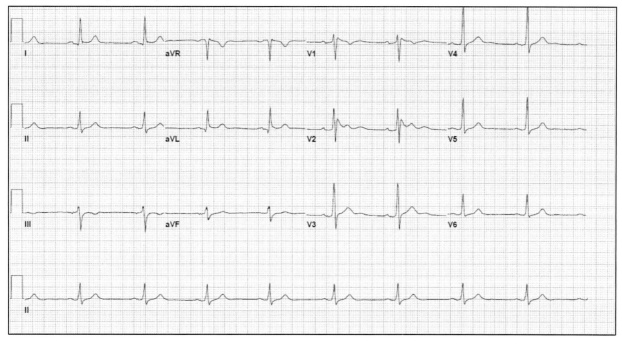

Brugada pattern type II, saddle-back-type

<u>Rate</u>: 54 <u>Rhythm</u>: sinus <u>Axis</u>: normal <u>Intervals</u>: normal <u>Ischemia</u>: none

What's the disposition and management?

The Brugada type II, or saddle-back pattern can be see here. This pattern is not diagnostic of the Brugada syndrome, but if the type I, or coved-type, pattern is unmasked in the electrophysiology lab by administration of sodium channel blockers (e.g. ajmaline), then the Brugada syndrome is diagnosed and an implantable defibrillator is warranted. This patient should be admitted for an electrophysiologic study to attempt to provoke the type I pattern. Type III is no longer considered in Brugada syndrome.[51] Type II Brugada can often look similar to an incomplete right bundle branch block (iRBBB), and certain measurements can be made on the ST angle to help differentiate.[52] Suffice it to say, with a true type II Brugada pattern, the r' wave in V1 and V2 is broad, rounded, and generally of low voltage with a slow descent, compared to that of an iRBBB, which is pointed.

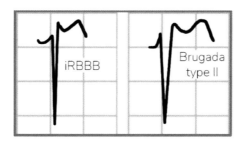

#3 – 45 yo F p/w dyspnea

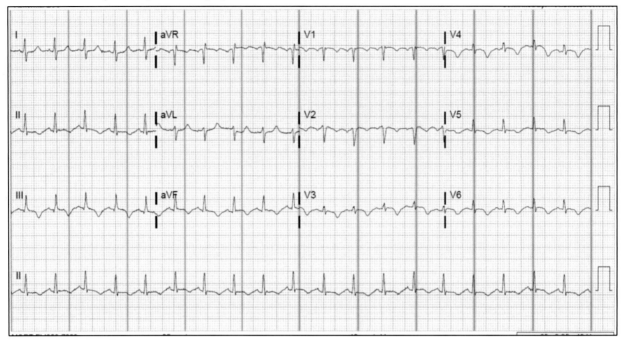

Rate: _____ Rhythm: _____ Axis: _____ Intervals: _____ Ischemia: _____

What is the next best step in management given hemodynamic instability?

What other ECG findings suggest the same diagnosis?

#3 – 45 yo F p/w dyspnea

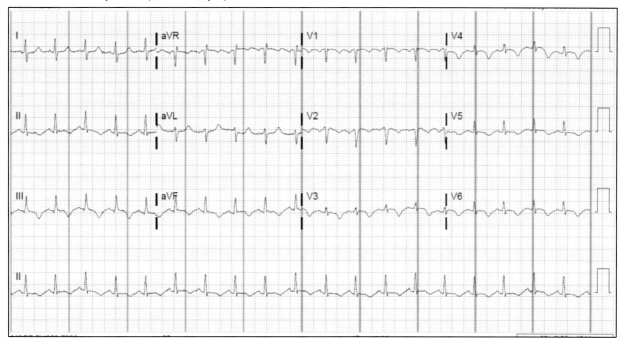

Pulmonary embolism, T-wave inversions

Rate: 114 Rhythm: sinus tachycardia Axis: normal Intervals: prolonged QT
Ischemia: diffuse T wave inversions

What is the next best step in management given hemodynamic instability?

If hemodynamically unstable, thrombolytics should be administered. No dosing regimen is clearly superior, but alteplase (50 – 100 mg given over 90 to 120 minutes) or tenecteplase (0.5 mg/kg bolus) has the most support.[53–56] There's lots of controversy surrounding administration of thrombolytics in patients with sub-massive pulmonary emboli, but hemodynamic instability makes the decision easier.

What other ECG findings suggest the same diagnosis?

Tachycardia, S1Q3T3, tall P wave in II, ST elevation in right-sided leads (aVR, V1, III), right axis deviation, new right bundle branch block, new incomplete right bundle branch block, and T wave inversions especially in the inferior and right-sided precordial leads (II, III, aVF, V1, V2, and V3) have all been suggested as right heart strain patterns.

#4 – 63 yo F p/w dyspnea

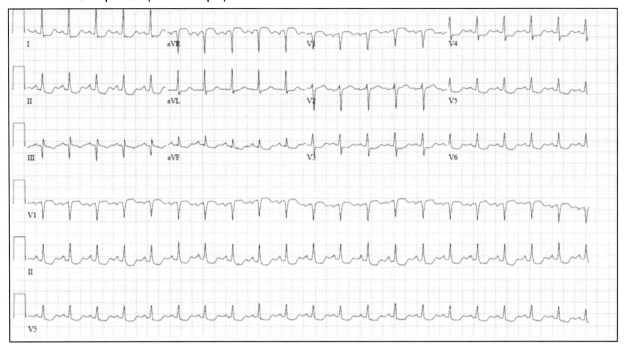

Rate: _____ Rhythm: _____ Axis: _____ Intervals: _____ Ischemia: _____

What is the differential diagnosis?

#4 – 63 yo F p/w dyspnea

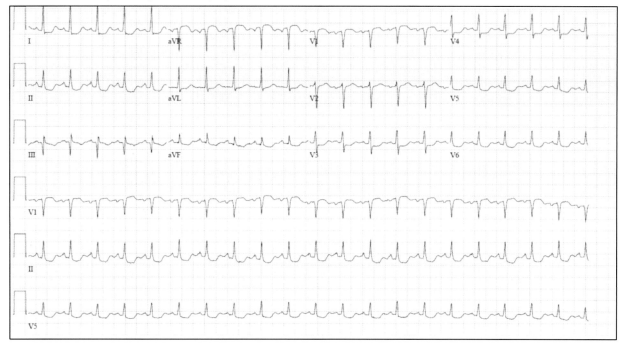

Pulmonary embolism, aVR ST elevation

Rate: 126 Rhythm: sinus Axis: normal Intervals: normal Ischemia: multilead ST depression with ST elevation in aVR

What is the differential diagnosis?

This case serves as a reminder that ECGs for patients with pulmonary emboli have variable appearances. This one had multilead ST depressions with aVR ST elevation. These findings resolved after systemic thrombolytics. This is also an excellent reminder of why aVR ST elevation is not a STEMI equivalent in terms of routine activation of emergent reperfusion, but rather nonspecific and suggestive of left main or multivessel disease in the right clinical context.

This pattern can result from nonocclusive causes such as baseline left ventricular hypertrophy or conditions that create a supply-demand mismatch such as acute blood loss, sepsis, respiratory failure, tachydysrhythmias, and aortic stenosis.[32] Although the mechanism is not clear, it is postulated that acute pulmonary embolism can lead to profound right and left ventricular ischemia, causing aVR-ST elevation, which can lead to a misdiagnosis of primary ischemic disease.[33]

#5 – 66 yo F p/w syncope

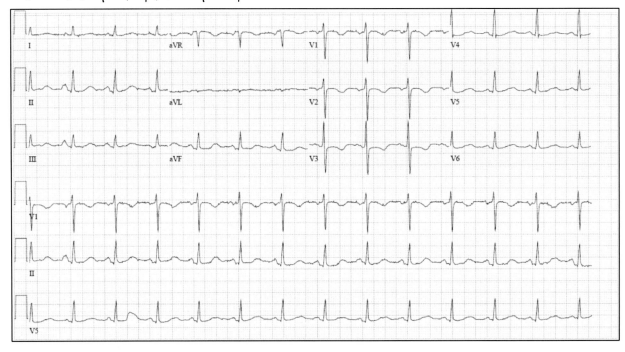

Rate: _____ Rhythm: _____ Axis: _____ Intervals: _____ Ischemia: _____

Which dysrhythmia is this patient at risk for?

What conditions can cause this ECG finding?

How would you manage this patient if she decompensated?

#5 – 66 yo F p/w syncope

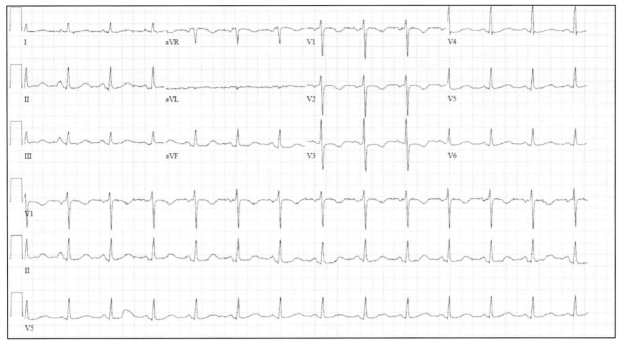

Prolonged QT

Rate: 84 Rhythm: sinus Axis: normal Intervals: prolonged QT Ischemia: slight ST depression and T wave inversions in V2/V3

Which dysrhythmia is this patient at risk for?

Torsades de Pointes due to early afterdepolarizations/triggered activity during the repolarization phase (R on T phenomenon).[57] It's worth noting that the QT correction formulas (e.g. Bazett's formula) are not very good outside a normal heart rate range, and that data supporting the use of a QT nomogram is emerging.[58,59]

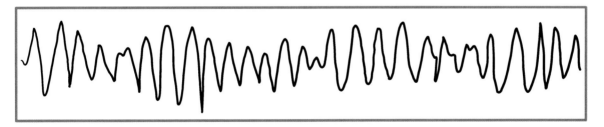

Torsades de Pointes

Measuring the QT can be challenging, and many different methods exist. One simple method is the "half the RR" rule – the QT interval is prolonged if it occupies more than half the R-R interval. The "half the RR" rule is a conservative estimate at normal and tachycardic rates, but perhaps a better option at bradycardic rates is an absolute cut-off of 485 ms.[59]

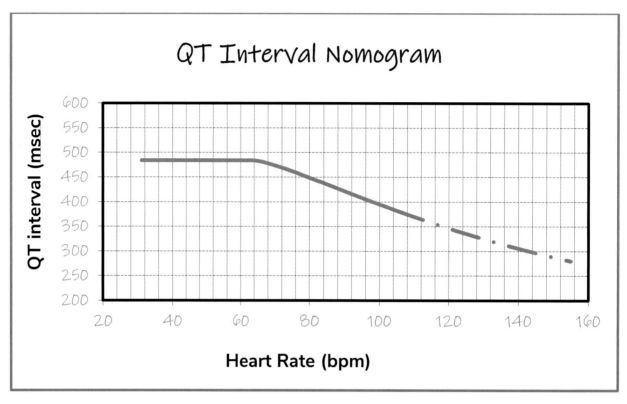

Derived from a database of toxicologic overdoses, the QT nomogram may provide a more reliable means of determining risk for Torsades de Pointes.[58]

What conditions can cause this ECG finding?

Causes of long QT include congenital cardiac ion channel mutations (i.e. Na or K channelopathies), electrolyte imbalance (i.e. hypokalemia, hypomagnesemia, hypocalcemia), medications (e.g. amiodarone, tricyclic antidepressants, methadone, antibiotics, ondansetron, antipsychotics, and many, many others), hypothermia, and hypothyroidism.[60]

How would you manage this patient if she decompensated?

Empiric administration of 2 g $MgSO_4$ and consideration of overdrive pacing to at least 100 bpm (either chemical with isoproterenol or electrical via transvenous pacing). Overdrive pacing works because tachycardia is protective against early afterdepolarizations.[57] The QT interval is inversely proportional to the heart rate; therefore, at faster heart rates, the QT interval is shorter and there is less opportunity for "early afterdepolarizations" (term used to describe abnormal depolarization during phase 2 or phase 3 of the cardiac action potential).

#6 – 57 yo M c̄ h/o etoh found down

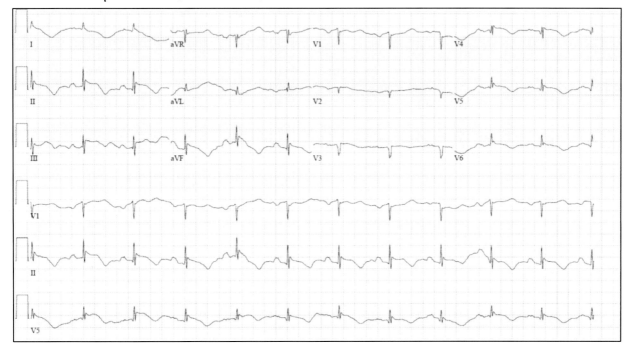

Rate: _____ Rhythm: _____ Axis: _____ Intervals: _____ Ischemia: _____

What environmental emergency does this patient have?

#6 – 57 yo M c̄ h/o etoh found down

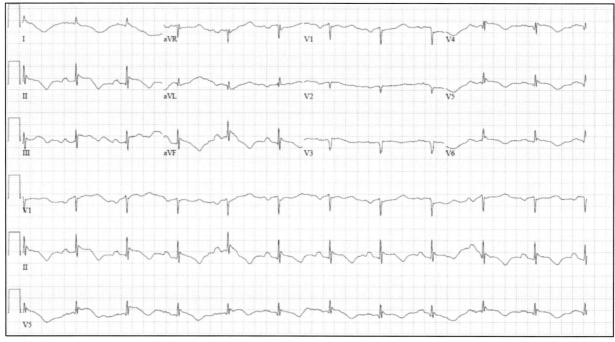

Hypothermia

<u>Rate</u>: 72 <u>Rhythm</u>: sinus <u>Axis</u>: normal <u>Intervals</u>: prolonged QT <u>Ischemia</u>: diffuse T wave inversions

What environmental emergency does this patient have?

Hypothermia, as evidenced by J waves, or Osborn waves. Hypothermia can also cause bradycardia, a prolonged QT, and motion artifact from shivering (this patient was paralyzed and intubated).[61] The T wave inversions and prolonged QT are likely explained by increased intracranial pressure from a pontine hemorrhage discovered on CT imaging (see next case for further explanation of this phenomenon known as "cerebral T waves").

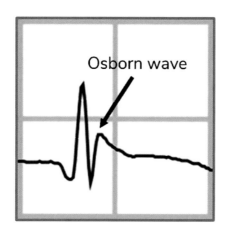

Osborn wave

#7 – 77 yo M p/w altered mental status

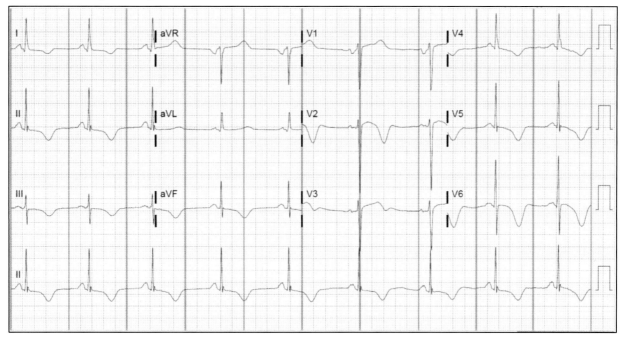

Rate: _____   Rhythm: _____   Axis: _____   Intervals: _____   Ischemia: _____

What are the next best steps in management?

#7 – 77 yo M p/w altered mental status

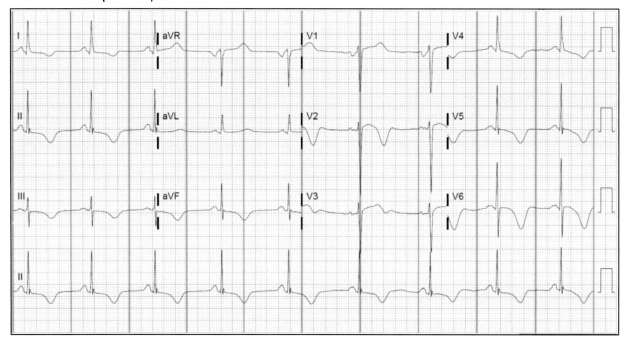

Cerebral T waves

Rate: 54   Rhythm: sinus bradycardia   Axis: normal   Intervals: prolonged QT   Ischemia: diffuse deep and symmetric T wave inversions

What are the next best steps in management?

The large T wave inversions are so-called "cerebral T waves" due to increased intracranial pressure as a result of intracranial hemorrhage. Cerebral T waves are likely the result of a sympathetic surge causing repolarization abnormalities. Cerebral T waves are rare and generally resolve over time.[62,63] The next best steps in management include airway management, elevating the head of the bead, aggressive blood pressure lowering, hyperosmolar therapy, and emergent neurosurgical consultation.

Unit 6

Ventricular Preexcitation
Causes of Sudden Cardiac Death
Repolarization Abnormalities
Myocardial Infarction and Conduction Disturbances
Low Voltage

#1 – 29 yo F p/w palpitations

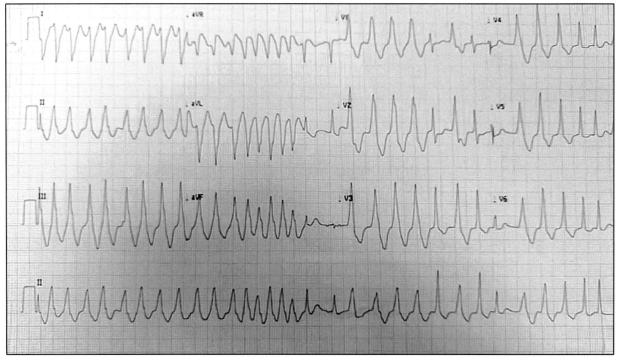

Rate: _____ Rhythm: _____ Axis: _____ Intervals: _____ Ischemia: _____

What triad of findings would you expect to see on the baseline resting ECG?

Assuming this patient is stable, what is the next best step in management?

What type of medications should be avoided?

#1 – 29 yo F p/w palpitations

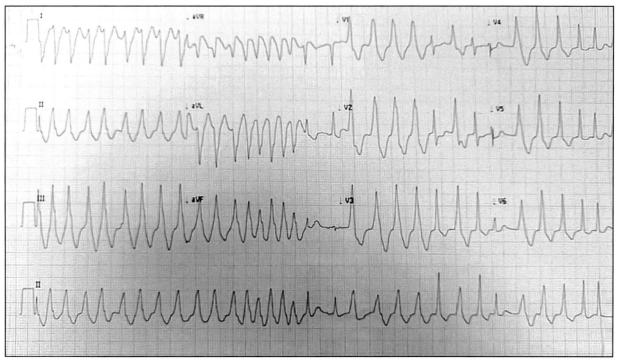

Atrial fibrillation with Wolf-Parkinson-White

Rate: 200 Rhythm: irregularly irregular Axis: right axis deviation Intervals: inconsistent QRS morphology Ischemia: n/a

What triad of findings would you expect to see on the baseline resting ECG?

This is an example of atrial fibrillation in a patient with Wolf-Parkinson-White (WPW). The QRS morphology is inconsistent owing to the variable transmission of signals from the atria to the ventricles. Normally, the atrioventricular node serves as the "gatekeeper" for signals arising from the atria – it has a refractory period that does not allow ventricular rates much faster than about 190.[64] Accessory pathways have short refractory periods, therefore signals can be transmitted at much faster rates (R-R interval as low as 200 ms = 300 bpm).[2]

Assuming this patient is stable, what is the next best step in management?

Patients with WPW and atrial fibrillation are at risk for deterioration and should be cardioverted. Procainamide or electrical cardioversion are the best options.

What type of medications should be avoided?

Atrioventricular nodal blocking agents (e.g. beta blockers) should be avoided. If the atrioventricular node is blocked, the fibrillatory atrial signals will be transmitted indiscriminately via the accessory pathway, precipitating ventricular fibrillation.[64]

#2 – 43 yo M p/w syncope

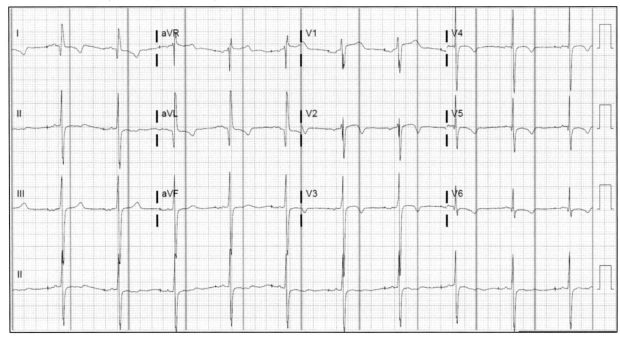

Rate: _____ Rhythm: _____ Axis: _____ Intervals: _____ Ischemia: _____

What electrocardiographic and physical exam finding suggests the diagnosis?

What are the treatment options?

What is the most appropriate disposition for this patient?

#2 – 43 yo M p/w syncope

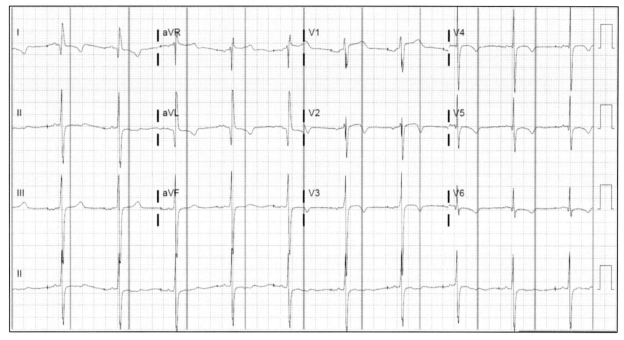

Hypertrophic cardiomyopathy

Rate: 60 Rhythm: atrial paced Axis: left axis deviation Intervals: normal Ischemia: anterolateral T wave inversions with high lateral Q waves (I and aVL)

What electrocardiographic and physical exam finding suggests the diagnosis?

The patient has hypertrophic cardiomyopathy, the most common cause of sudden cardiac death among individuals < 40 years of age.[57] A systolic murmur along the left sternal border that is potentiated with maneuvers that reduce preload (e.g. Valsalva) and attenuated with maneuvers that increase afterload (e.g. squatting) is characteristic. ECG findings include left ventricular hypertrophy, T wave inversions (especially in lateral leads), and narrow Q waves (i.e. "dagger Q waves") in the lateral leads (I, aVL, V5, V6).[2,65]

Syncope Findings on ECG that you can't miss
1. Hypertrophic cardiomyopathy
2. Brugada
3. Wolf - Parkinson - White
4. Long QT
5. Arrhythmogenic right ventricular cardiomyopathy

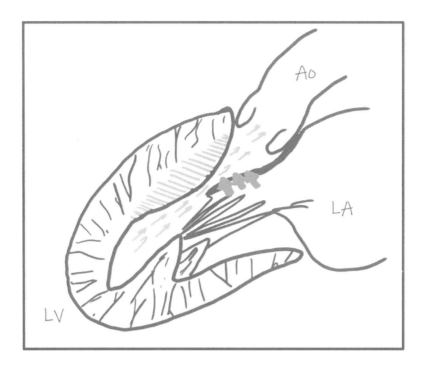

Depiction of outflow obstruction of hypertrophic cardiomyopathy. The anterior leaflet of the mitral valve (red arrows) moves towards the hypertrophied septum (blue lines), creating an outflow obstruction. LA, left atrium; Ao, aorta; LV, left ventricle.

What are the treatment options?

Treatment options include beta blockers, amiodarone, implantable cardioverter-defibrillator placement, surgical myomectomy, and septal ablation.[65] Atrioventricular nodal blockers work by prolonging diastolic filling, making outflow obstruction less likely.

What is the most appropriate disposition for this patient?

If patient has good follow up and is reliable, referral to cardiology as outpatient for echocardiogram and ambulatory monitoring, otherwise admit for expedited work-up.

#3 – 53 yo M p/w chest pain, currently chest pain-free

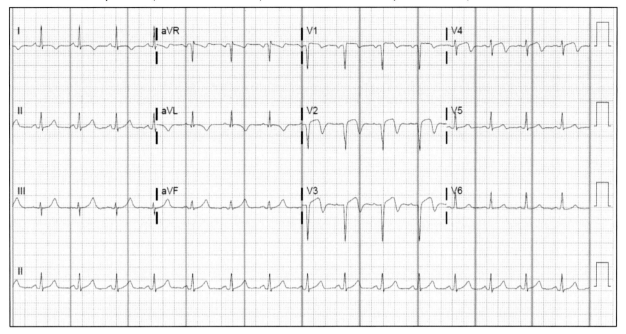

Rate: _____ Rhythm: _____ Axis: _____ Intervals: _____ Ischemia: _____

Is emergent reperfusion indicated?

What are the initial critical actions?

#3 – 53 yo M p/w chest pain, currently chest pain-free

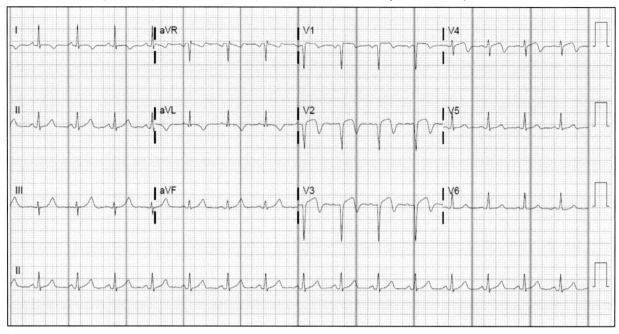

Wellens syndrome

Rate: 90 Rhythm: sinus Axis: normal Intervals: normal Ischemia: biphasic T waves in anterior precordial leads

Is emergent reperfusion indicated?

No, but the clinical context and ECG findings suggest a critical stenosis of the left anterior descending artery and urgent catheterization is warranted. Wellens syndrome comes in two electrocardiographic varieties – biphasic T waves (up then down) or deeply inverted and symmetric T waves in the anterior precordial leads (V1-V3).

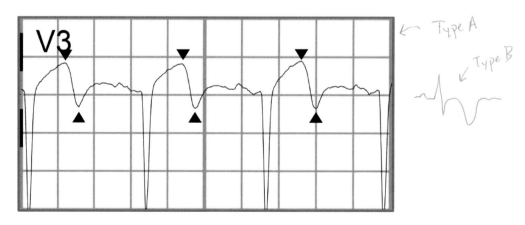

Biphasic T waves (▼▲) with terminal negativity (▲) in V3.

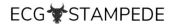

The syndrome requires these ECG findings in a patient that is chest pain free. If the patient develops chest pain and the T waves "pseudonormalize" (i.e. become upright), complete occlusion is suggested.[66] Wellens syndrome represents a special category of high-risk acute coronary syndrome that should have an urgent catheterization planned with the cardiologist. This patient was found to have a 95% critical stenosis of the proximal left anterior descending artery. Patients in whom Wellens syndrome is a consideration should not get a stress test given the risk of a large anterior myocardial infarction.

What are the initial critical actions?

Treat these patients as though they have acute coronary syndrome per your institutional protocol – i.e. aspirin, P2Y12 inhibitors, anticoagulation, etc…

#4 – 67 yo M p/w chest pain

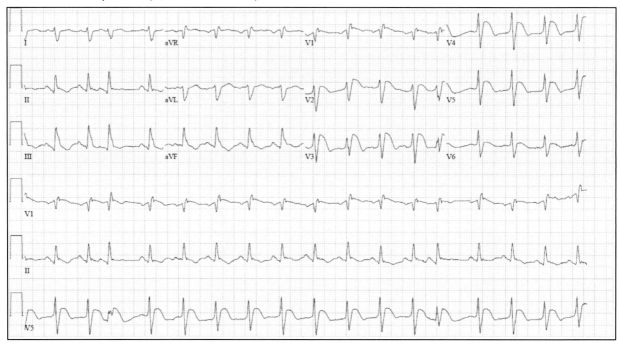

Rate: _____ Rhythm: _____ Axis: _____ Intervals: _____ Ischemia: _____

Is emergent reperfusion indicated?

What findings suggest a poorer prognosis?

#4 – 67 yo M p/w chest pain

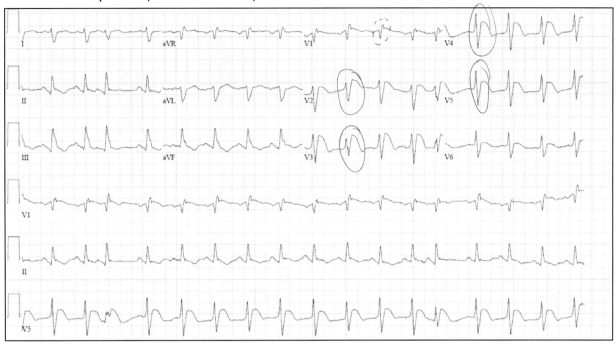

Anterior STEMI and bifascicular block
bifascicular block

Rate: 96 Rhythm: sinus Axis: right axis deviation Intervals: prolonged QT, wide QRS
Ischemia: ST elevation in anterior precordial leads

Is emergent reperfusion indicated?

Yes, this patient had a left anterior descending artery occlusion. Remember, even subtle ST elevation in the anterior leads (i.e. V1-3) in the presence of right bundle branch block (RBBB) is abnormal. Normally, RBBB has slight ST depression or isoelectric ST segments in the anterior precordial leads, but never ST elevations.[9]

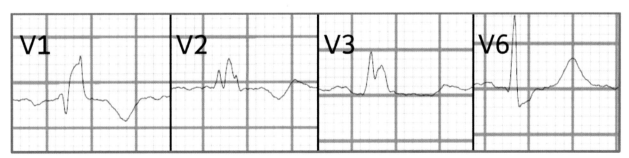

Typical right bundle branch morphology in V1, V2, V3, and V6

What findings suggest a poorer prognosis?

Patients with right bundle branch blocks and acute myocardial infarctions (with or without fascicular blocks) have poorer prognoses.[20,21]

#5 – 29 yo F p/w dyspnea

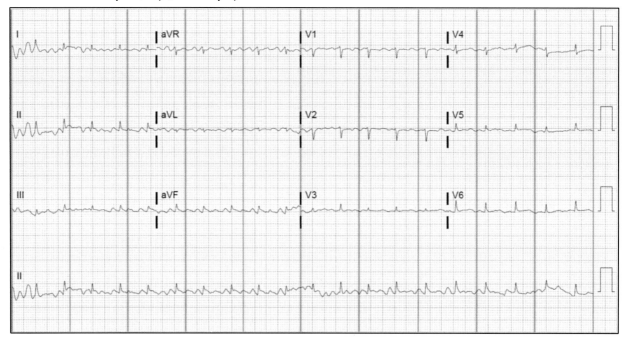

Rate: _____ Rhythm: _____ Axis: _____ Intervals: _____ Ischemia: _____

What is the definition of low voltage?

What is the differential diagnosis for low voltage?

#5 – 29 yo F p/w dyspnea

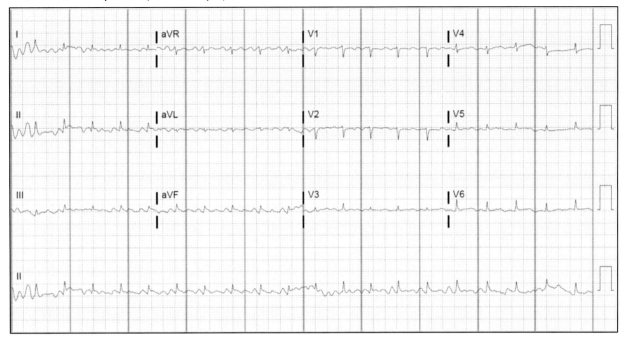

Low voltage

Rate: 122   Rhythm: sinus   Axis: normal   Intervals: normal   Ischemia: none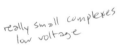

really small complexes low voltage

What is the definition of low voltage?

The traditional definition of low voltage is QRS amplitudes less than 5 mm in all limb leads or less than 10 mm in all precordial leads.[67]   *this EKG meets both*

What is the differential diagnosis for low voltage?

The differential for low voltage can be conceptualized by considering two categories: cardiac abnormalities resulting in diminished impulse generation and increased impedance related to attenuating substances between the heart and surface leads (fluid, air, or adipose). Cardiac causes include prior infarcts, infiltrative cardiomyopathies like amyloidosis, and hypothyroidism. Extracardiac causes include pericardial processes like pericardial effusion or constrictive calcific pericarditis, chronic obstructive pulmonary disease, pleural effusion, subcutaneous or mediastinal emphysema, and obesity. The combination of low voltage and bradycardia should raise the concern for hypothyroidism/myxedema.[60]

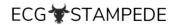

Increased Impedance	Decreased Impulse Generation

Pericardial
  Effusion
  Constrictive pericarditis
  Pneumopericardium
Thoracic
  Intra-pleural
    Pneumothorax
    Pleural effusion
  Pulmonary
    COPD
    Pulmonary edema
  Mediastinum
    Pneumomediastinum
Soft tissue
  Peripheral edema
  Obesity
	Prior myocardial infarction
	Infiltrative cardiomyopathy (amyloidosis, sarcoidosis)
	Myocarditis
	Hypothyroidism

Causes of electrocardiographic low voltage.

This patient had a large pericardial effusion causing pericardial tamponade and underwent an emergent pericardiocentesis with hemodynamic improvement. Always consider cardiac tamponade when the ECG shows low voltage and tachycardia.

Unit 7

Conduction Disturbances
Electrolyte Derangements

#1 – 66 yo M p/w weakness

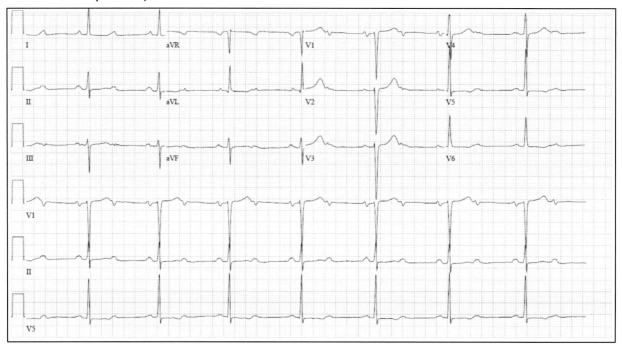

Rate: _____ Rhythm: _____ Axis: _____ Intervals: _____ Ischemia: _____

What is the location of the conduction block?

What is the definitive treatment for this patient?

Which atrioventricular blocks portend worse prognoses?

#1 – 66 yo M p/w weakness

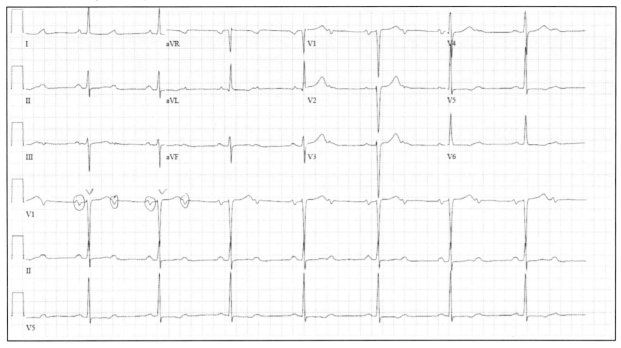

2:1 atrioventricular block

Rate: atrial 84, ventricular 42   Rhythm: 2:1 atrioventricular block   Axis: left axis deviation   Intervals: normal QRS and QT   Ischemia: none

What is the location of the conduction block?

Trick question. This is a 2:1 atrioventricular block, so it is impossible to know whether it is Mobitz I (nodal) or Mobitz II (infranodal) based on the surface ECG. It was later confirmed to be infranodal when a subsequent ECG showed Mobitz II.

What is the definitive treatment for this patient?

This patient needs a pacemaker. A 2:1 atrioventricular block should be presumed to be infranodal and, therefore, more likely to progress to complete heart block with an unreliable escape rhythm originating in the distal Purkinje fibers.

Which atrioventricular blocks portend worse prognoses?

Conduction defects at the atrioventricular node result in delayed or intermittent conduction through the atrioventricular node; those below the atrioventricular node carry a worse prognosis because they are more likely to progress to complete heart block and less likely to have reliable escape rhythms.

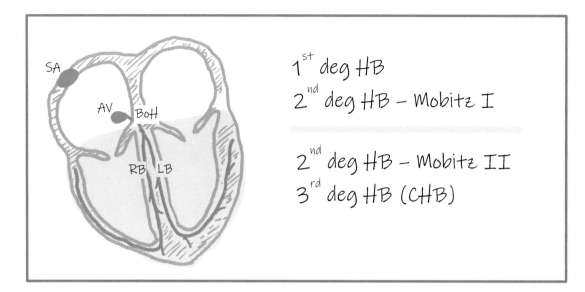

1ˢᵗ deg HB
2ⁿᵈ deg HB – Mobitz I

2ⁿᵈ deg HB – Mobitz II
3ʳᵈ deg HB (CHB)

Conduction defects above the blue line are typically the result of delayed or intermittent conduction through the atrioventricular node; those below the blue line are the result of conduction disease below the atrioventricular node and carry a worse prognosis. SA, sinoatrial node; AV, atrioventricular node; BoH, bundle of His; LB, left bundle; RB, right bundle; HB, heart block; CHB, complete heart block.

First degree atrioventricular block is represented by prolongation of the atrioventricular conduction time (PR interval) beyond 0.2 s, while every atrial impulse is conducted to the ventricle. First degree block usually suggests delayed conduction through the atrioventricular node, and is generally considered to be a benign phenomenon when not associated with other conduction deficits (i.e. right bundle branch block with a concomitant left anterior or posterior fascicular block, a so-called "bifascicular block").[9,19]

Third degree atrioventricular block (complete heart block, CHB) occurs when there is complete atrioventricular dissociation (i.e. failure of conduction between the atria and the ventricles). With CHB, the level of escape rhythm determines not only the heart rate, but also the reliability of the rhythm. For example, when the atrioventricular node is diseased and fails to conduct, a junctional escape rhythm (at the level of the bundle of His) emerges which usually produces a more reliable rate between 40 and 60 BPM. However, when infrahisian conduction disease exists (i.e. below the bundle of His), the escape rhythms are ventricular in origin and tend to be slower, and less reliable.[8]

Second degree atrioventricular block occurs when there is intermittent atrioventricular conduction and can represent conduction deficits at the level of the atrioventricular node or at the infrahisian level. Electrocardiographically, it is characterized by a

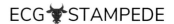

progressively prolonging PR interval until conduction from the atria to the ventricle fails. Second degree Mobitz type I blocks are often asymptomatic and seen it active, healthy patients without heart disease – it usually represents disease within the atrioventricular node itself, which is unlikely to progress to CHB.[3] However, second degree Mobitz type I block can indicate infrahisian conduction disease when accompanied by preexisting conduction disease (e.g. right bundle branch block, left bundle branch block, or bifascicular block).

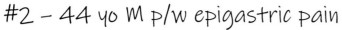

#2 – 44 yo M p/w epigastric pain

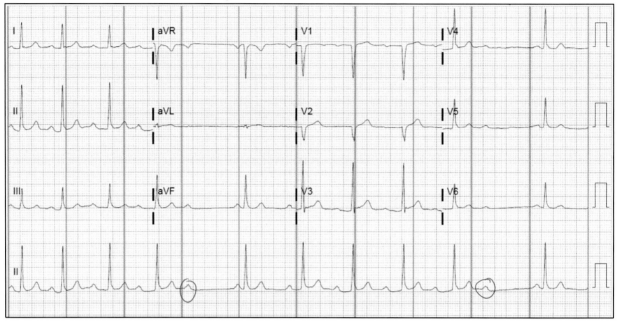

Rate: _____ Rhythm: _____ Axis: _____ Intervals: _____ Ischemia: _____

What are the causes of this rhythm?

What is the location of the conduction block?

What are the locations and expected rates of the intrinsic pacemakers?

What is the disposition?

#2 – 44 yo M p/w epigastric pain

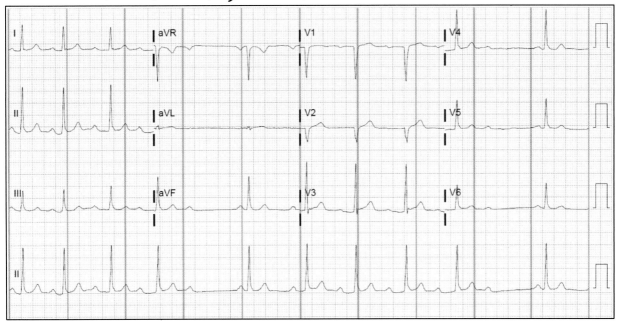

Second degree heart block, Mobitz I (Wenckebach)

Rate: atrial 72, ventricular 60   Rhythm: 6:5 Mobitz I   Axis: normal   Intervals: normal QRS and QT, progressively prolonging PR   Ischemia: none

What are the causes of this rhythm?

Causes include atrioventricular nodal blocking drugs (e.g. beta blockers, calcium channel blockers, digitalis), inferior myocardial infarction, increased vagal tone.[2]

What is the location of the conduction block?

Mobitz I is usually a reversible conduction block at the atrioventricular node.

What are the locations and expected rates of the intrinsic pacemakers?

The upper limits of normal for intrinsic pacemakers are: sinus node, 100 bpm; atria, 100 bpm; common His bundle 60 bpm; bundle branches 50 bpm. Rates exceeding these arbitrary upper limits are considered accelerated (e.g. an accelerated junctional rhythm exceeds a rate of 60 bpm). Atrial and ventricular muscle cells and atrioventricular nodal cells do not have pace-making capabilities.[2]

What is the disposition?

The patient can be safely discharged if asymptomatic and no evidence of block progression. However, with an atrial rate of 70, 3:2 or 4:3 block (ventricular rate 46 bpm and 51 bpm, respectively) may be sufficient to make an elderly patient symptomatic.

#3 – 85 yo M presents status post vehicle accident

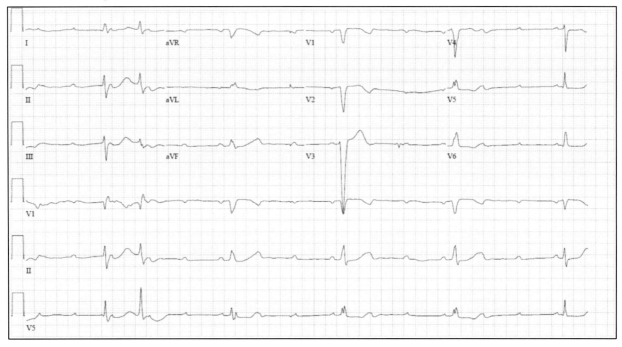

Rate: _____ Rhythm: _____ Axis: _____ Intervals: _____ Ischemia: _____

What are the causes of this rhythm?

What is the location of the conduction block?

What is the treatment?

#3 – 85 yo M presents status post vehicle accident

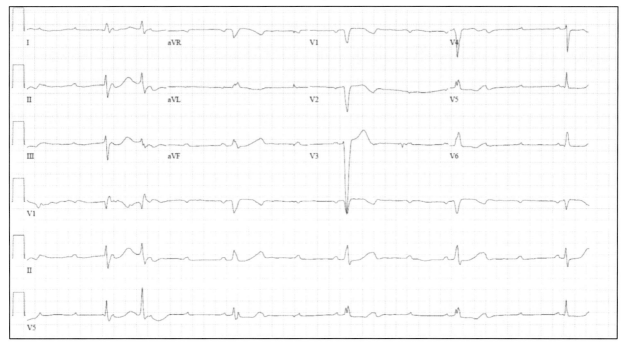

Second degree Mobitz II, 3:1 atrioventricular block

Rate: atrial 90 ventricular 30 Rhythm: 3:1 Mobitz II Axis: normal Intervals: QRS widening Ischemia: none

What are the causes of this rhythm?

Atrioventricular block is cause by structural damage to the conducting system (e.g. infarction, fibrosis, necrosis).

What is the location of the conduction block?

Mobitz II is usually irreversible infranodal damage, it is almost always preceded by a bundle-branch block pattern for the conducted beats, with the non-conducted beats resulting from intermittent block in the other bundle branch. Continuous block in the other bundle branch results in syncope or heart failure if ventricular escape occurs, and sudden death if there is no ventricular escape. Narrow escape complexes always represent atrioventricular nodal blocks.[2,8]

What is the treatment?

If the patient is symptomatic, pacing should be attempted. Atropine can potentially worsen infranodal blocks by sending more electrical stress through an already failing conduction system.[8] If permanent pacing is not immediately planned, transvenous pacing should be considered given the danger of progression.

#4 – 62 yo M p/w fatigue

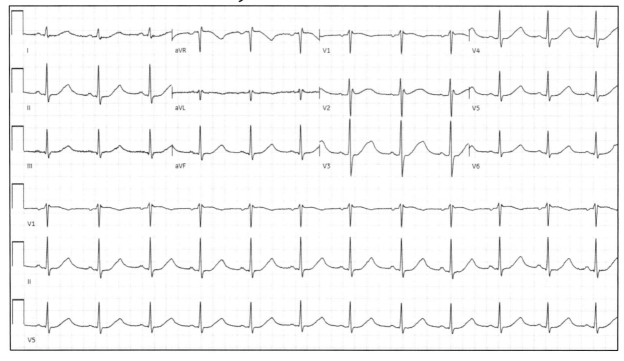

Rate: _____ Rhythm: _____ Axis: _____ Intervals: _____ Ischemia: _____

What common electrolyte disturbance is responsible for the ECG abnormalities?

#4 – 62 yo M p/w fatigue

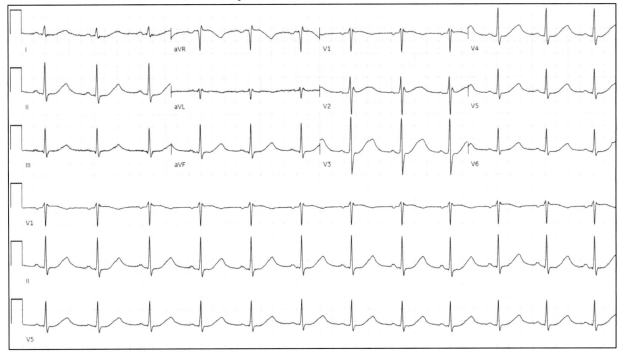

Prolonged QT due to hypokalemia

<u>Rate</u>: 72 <u>Rhythm</u>: sinus <u>Axis</u>: normal <u>Intervals</u>: prolonged QT <u>Ischemia</u>: none

What common electrolyte disturbance is responsible for the ECG abnormalities?

Electrolytes effect different parts of the action potential and, therefore, tend to effect specific intervals as shown below. This patient was severely hypokalemic. The prolonged QT interval resolved after potassium replacement.

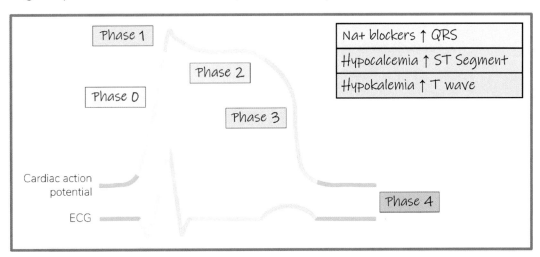

See Unit 4, case # 3 for further explanation of electrolyte disturbances and their effects on the ECG.

#5 – 50 yo M p/w R foot pain

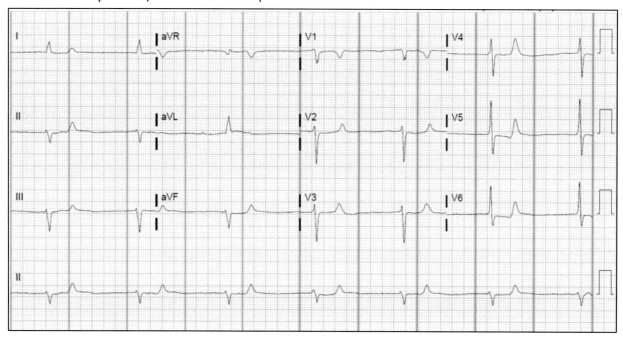

Rate: _____ Rhythm: _____ Axis: _____ Intervals: _____ Ischemia: _____

What is the treatment?

With this condition, what three ECG features predict adverse outcomes and what is the expected progression of ECG changes?

#5 – 50 yo M p/w R foot pain

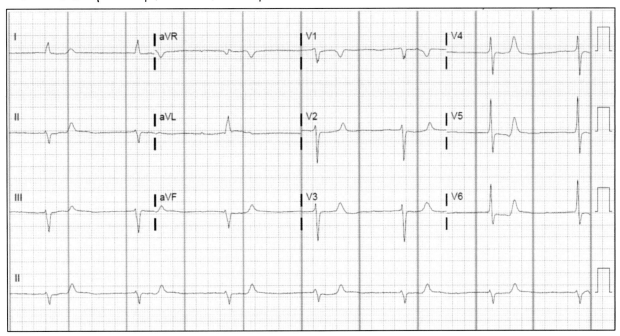

Hyperkalemia, junctional rhythm and peaked T waves

<u>Rate</u>: 42 <u>Rhythm</u>: junctional <u>Axis</u>: left axis deviation <u>Intervals</u>: slightly widened QRS, prolonged QT, no PR interval <u>Ischemia</u>: ST depressions inf V4, V5, & V6

What is the treatment?

Membrane stabilizers include calcium and hypertonic saline. Intracellular potassium shifters include insulin/glucose, beta-agonists, and sodium bicarbonate in acidotic patients. Potassium eliminators include loop diuretics and kayexalate. New medications to promote gastrointestinal excretion hold promise (patiromer and sodium zirconium cyclosilicate).[43]

With this condition, what three ECG features predict adverse outcomes and what is the expected progression of ECG changes?

1) Bradycardia < 50 bpm
2) QRS > 110 ms
3) Junctional rhythm

Notice that peaked T waves were not found to predict acute adverse outcomes.[44]

Serum Potassium[43]	Potential ECG Changes	Morphology
5.5-6.5 mEq/L	Tall, peaked T waves with narrow base	Peaked T wave
	QT interval shortening	
	ST-segment depression	
6.5-8.0 mEq/L	Peaked T waves	Blunted P wave Prolonged PR Wide QRS
	PR-interval prolongation	
	P wave decreased amplitude or disappearance	
	QRS widening	Absent P wave
	R-wave amplification	
> 8.0 mEq/L	P-wave absence	
	QRS widening	Sine wave
	Intraventricular/fascicular/bundle branch blocks	
	Sine wave	

This table shows the expected electrocardiographic changes with given serum potassium levels. It is important to note that potassium-related electrocardiographic changes do not always follow this progression.

Unit 8

Conduction Disturbances
Atrial Enlargement
Electrolyte Derangements

#1 – 51 yo M p/w chest pain and dizziness

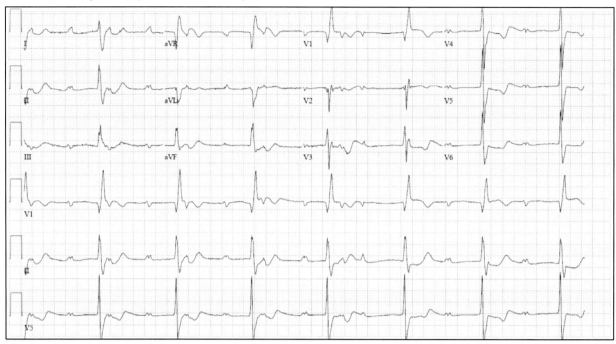

Rate: _____ Rhythm: _____ Axis: _____ Intervals: _____ Ischemia: _____

What is the location of the conduction block?

What is the definitive treatment for this patient?

(See baseline ECG on next page)

#1 – 51 yo M p/w chest pain and dizziness (baseline ECG)

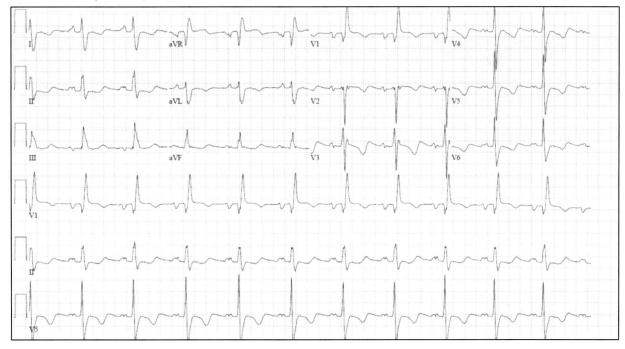

Rate: _____ Rhythm: _____ Axis: _____ Intervals: _____ Ischemia: _____

#1 – 51 yo M p/w chest pain and dizziness

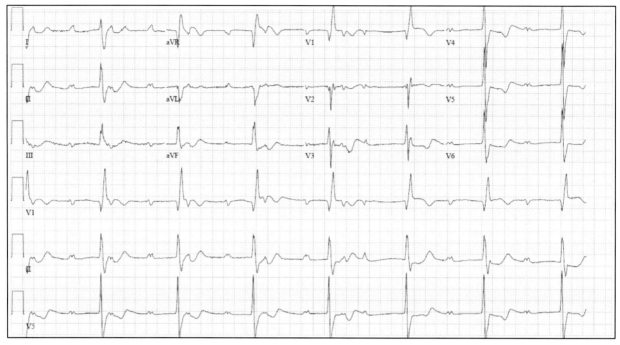

Complete heart block

Rate: atrial 84, ventricular 42 Rhythm: likely junctional escape Axis: right axis deviation Intervals: wide QRS Ischemia: none

What is the location of the conduction block?

The baseline ECG shows trifascicular disease (right bundle branch block, left posterior fascicular block, and first-degree atrioventricular block). The block could be in the atrioventricular node because the QRS morphology is the same as in the baseline ECG, suggesting that a junctional escape rhythm is conducting through the single remaining fascicle (i.e. left anterior fascicle). The rhythm could also represent ventricular escape. An electrophysiology study would be needed to determine the exact location of the block. See the next page for a more detailed explanation of block location and escape rhythms.

What is the definitive treatment for this patient?

This patient needs a permanent pacemaker. If unstable, the patient should be externally paced or paced with a transvenous pacemaker at the bedside.

#1 – 51 yo M p/w chest pain and dizziness (baseline ECG)

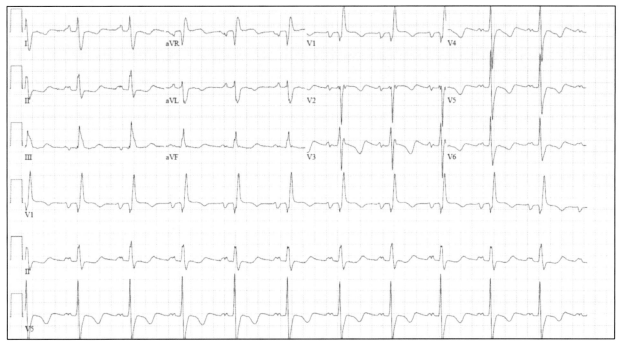

Left atrial enlargement, trifascicular block

<u>Rate</u>: 66   <u>Rhythm</u>: sinus   <u>Axis</u>: right axis deviation   <u>Intervals</u>: wide QRS, prolonged PR
<u>Ischemia</u>: none

Blocks can occur anywhere from the atrioventricular node to the distal infranodal conduction system (i.e. Purkinje network). The atrioventricular node does not have intrinsic pace-making ability like the rest of the His-Purkinje network, and blocks of the common His bundle are exceptionally rare; therefore, patients with complete heart block often have pre-existing conduction disturbances (e.g. bi or trifascicular disease) and complete heart block results following an insult to the remaining fascicle. When blocks of the infranodal trifascicular conduction system occur, a wide complex "ventricular" escape rhythm arises from the distal Purkinje fibers. Alternatively, an insult to the atrioventricular node can render it non-conducting, also resulting in complete (*nodal*) heart block. When complete *nodal* heart block occurs, a narrow complex "junctional" escape rhythm arises from the common His bundle.

Although the complex on the presenting ECG is wide, this patient could have complete *nodal* heart block with a junctional escape rhythm resulting from a diseased atrioventricular node. The wide complex escape rhythm could be explained by the pre-existing right bundle branch block seen in the baseline ECG. An electrophysiology study would be needed to determine the exact location of the block.

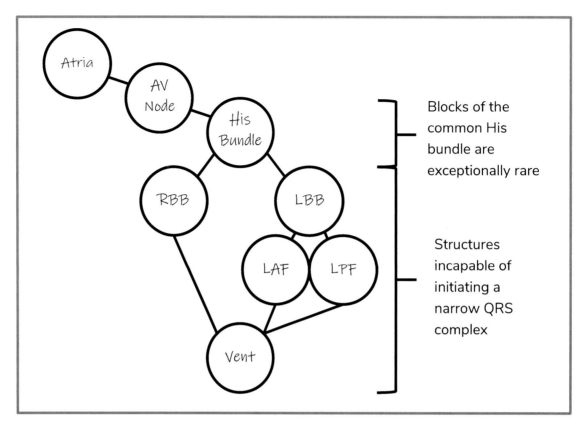

Schematic of the conducting system from the atria to the ventricles.[2] AV, atrioventricular; RBB, right bundle branch; LBB, left bundle branch; LAF, left anterior fascicle; LPF, left posterior fascicle.

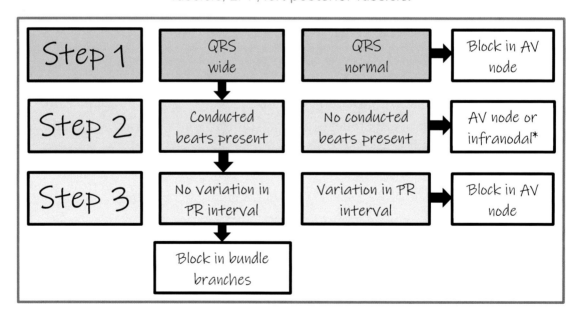

Algorithm to aid in the determination of the location of the block (i.e. nodal vs infranodal) when interpreting heart blocks.[2] *Complete heart block, more information is needed to determine location. AV, atrioventricular.

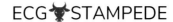

Atrial Enlargement

This patient also has signs of left atrial enlargement, or P-mitrale, with a wide and notched P wave in lead II. In general, atrial enlargement can be determined by analyzing the P waves in leads II and V1. The first half of the P wave represents right atrial depolarization, while the second half represents left atrial depolarization.

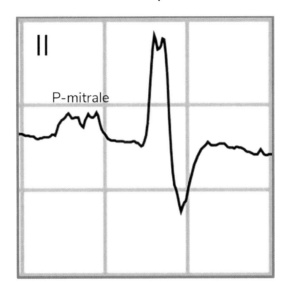

Lead II complex demonstrating left atrial enlargement, or P-mitrale. Note the notched and wide appearance of the P wave.

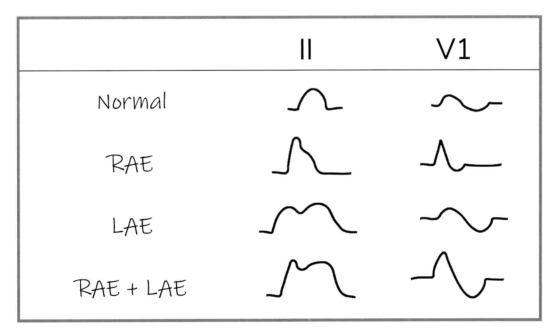

P wave morphologies for atrial enlargement in leads II and V1.[2] RAE, right atrial enlargement; LAE, left atrial enlargement.

#2 – 61 yo M p/w bradycardia

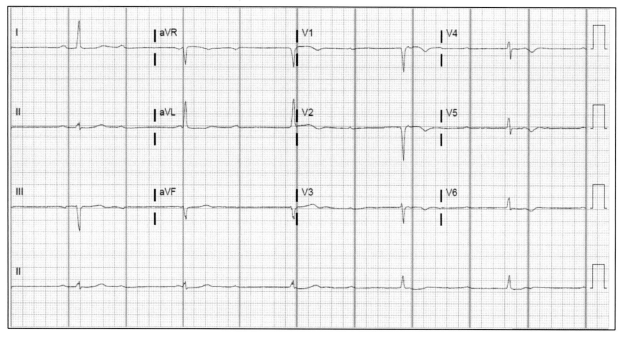

Rate: _____ Rhythm: _____ Axis: _____ Intervals: _____ Ischemia: _____

What is the location of the conduction block?

Would atropine work?

What is the definitive treatment for this patient?

#2 – 61 yo M p/w bradycardia

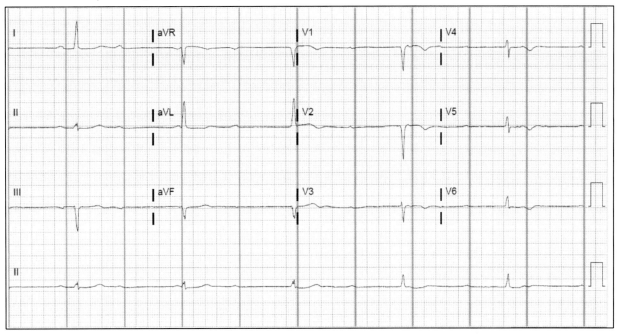

Complete heart block with a junctional escape rhythm

<u>Rate</u>: atrial 60, ventricular 30   <u>Rhythm</u>: junctional escape   <u>Axis</u>: left axis deviation

<u>Intervals</u>: normal QRS and QT   <u>Ischemia</u>: Anterolateral T wave inversions

What is the location of the conduction block?

The QRS is narrow, therefore the escape rhythm is junctional, and the location of the block must be nodal (even despite the slow junctional escape rhythm).

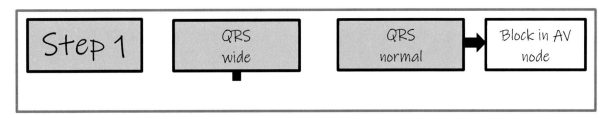

Step 1 of the algorithm from Unit 1, case #8.

Would atropine work?

Atropine improves nodal conduction and, therefore, may be helpful in this scenario.[8] Atropine is potentially harmful when the location of the block is infranodal.

What is the definitive treatment for this patient?

This patient needs a permanent pacemaker. If unstable, the patient should be externally paced or paced with a transvenous pacemaker at the bedside.

#3 – 69 yo F p/w slurred speech

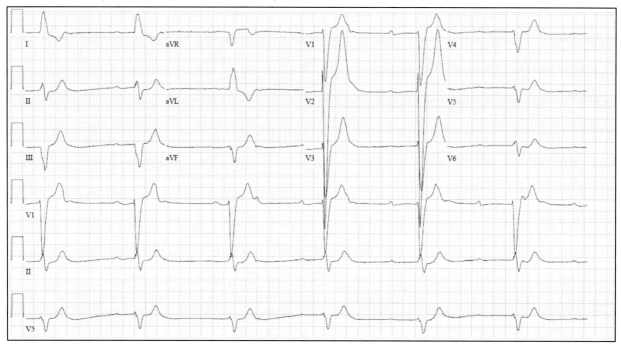

Rate: _____ Rhythm: _____ Axis: _____ Intervals: _____ Ischemia: _____

What is the location of the conduction block?

Would atropine work?

What is the definitive treatment for this patient?

#3 – 69 yo F p/w slurred speech

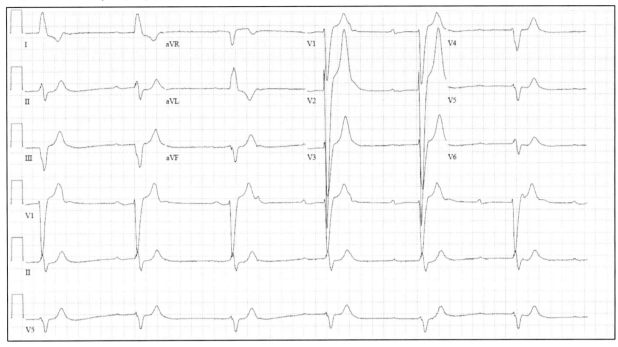

Complete heart block with a ventricular escape rhythm

<u>Rate</u>: atrial 72, ventricular 36 <u>Rhythm</u>: ventricular escape <u>Axis</u>: left axis deviation
<u>Intervals</u>: wide QRS <u>Ischemia</u>: none

What is the location of the conduction block?

There is a ventricular escape rhythm (owing to the slow rate < 40 bpm and wide QRS complex), so the location of the block is most likely infranodal.

Would atropine work?

Atropine is not likely to work and is not recommended in this scenario. Atropine can potentially worsen infranodal blocks by sending more electrical stress through an already failing conduction system.[8]

What is the definitive treatment for this patient?

This patient needs a permanent pacemaker. If unstable, the patient should be externally paced or paced with a transvenous pacemaker at the bedside.

#4 – 58 yo M p/w chest pain

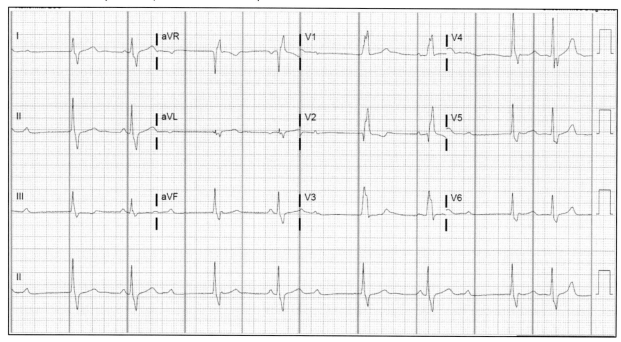

Rate: _____ Rhythm: _____ Axis: _____ Intervals: _____ Ischemia: _____

What is the location of the conduction block?

Would atropine work?

What is the definitive treatment for this patient?

(See prior ECG on next page)

#4 – 58 yo M p/w chest pain (ECG from 1 day prior)

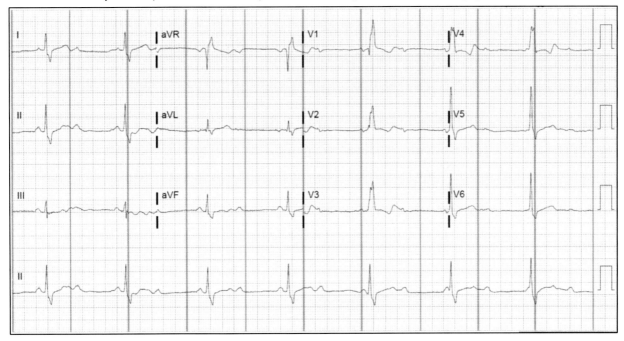

Rate: _____ Rhythm: _____ Axis: _____ Intervals: _____ Ischemia: _____

#4 – 58 yo M p/w chest pain

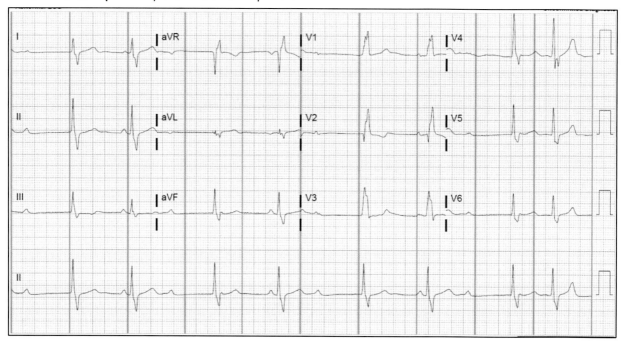

Second degree heart block (Mobitz I)

<u>Rate</u>: atrial 66, ventricular 48 <u>Rhythm</u>: 3:2 atrioventricular block <u>Axis</u>: normal
<u>Intervals</u>: wide QRS <u>Ischemia</u>: none

What is the location of the conduction block?

Mobitz I (Wenckebach) is characterized by progressive PR segment prolongation
followed by a non-conducted beat (leading to the appearance of "grouped" beats). It
is most often caused by increased vagal tone but can be caused by a diseased
atrioventricular node. It is often thought of as benign; however, as we see with this
case, Mobitz I can progress to complete heart block. This case highlights the
importance of clinical context when interpreting ECGs. If a young athlete is discovered
to have Mobitz I, there is little to no concern; however, in a 58-year-old with evidence
of conduction disease (e.g. right bundle branch block), Mobitz I can be quite
concerning.

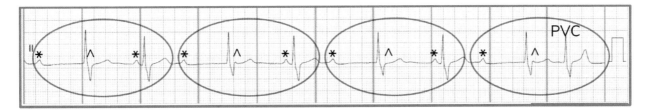

Ellipses demarcate the 3:2 conduction pattern. Conducted P waves are represented by an asterisk (*) and non-conducted by a carrot-top (^). The final beat is a premature ventricular complex (PVC), but could also be a premature junctional complex (PJC).

Would atropine work?

Atropine improves nodal conduction and, therefore, may be helpful in this scenario.[8]

#4 – 58 yo M p/w chest pain (ECG from 1 day prior)

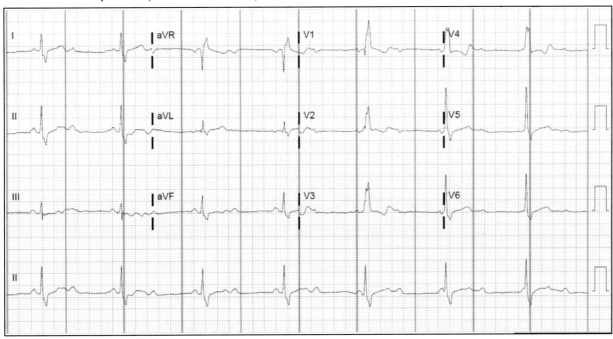

Complete heart block with junctional escape rhythm

Rate: atrial 84, ventricular 42 Rhythm: junctional escape Axis: normal Intervals: wide QRS Ischemia: none

At first glance, the P waves appear to be conducted; however, upon closer interrogation of the lead II rhythm strip, the PR interval is shortening. There is no electrophysiologic explanation for a shortening PR interval aside from atrioventricular dissociation (i.e. complete heart block).

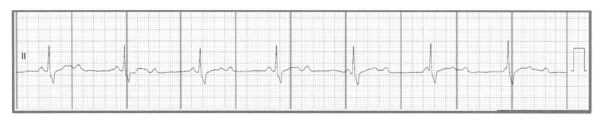

Rhythm strip demonstrating inconsistent and shortening PR interval. There is no electrophysiologic explanation for a shortening PR interval aside from atrioventricular dissociation (i.e. complete heart block).

Since the QRS morphology appears consistent with the patient's known right bundle branch block, and the ventricular rate is 42 bpm, the most likely escape rhythm is junctional, which tends to produce a rate between 40 and 60 bpm.

What is the definitive treatment for this patient?

This is complete *nodal* heart block, and a permanent pacemaker is indicated. If unstable, external or transvenous pacing should be pursued at the bedside.

#5 – 62 yo M p/w fatigue

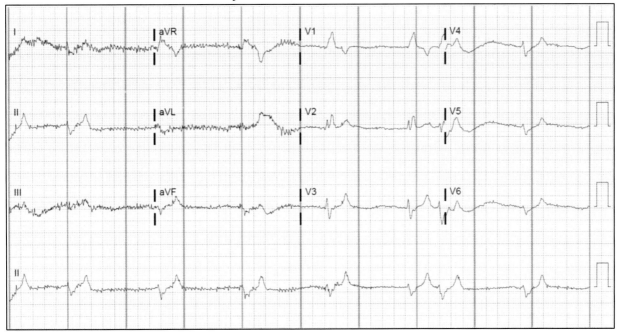

Rate: _____ Rhythm: _____ Axis: _____ Intervals: _____ Ischemia: _____

What is the rhythm?

What is the first line treatment?

#5 – 62 yo M p/w fatigue

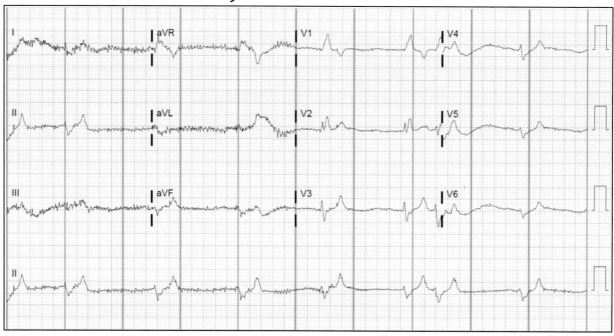

Hyperkalemia, wide QRS and peaked T waves

Rate: ventricular 48 Rhythm: unclear escape rhythm with ectopy Axis: left axis deviation Intervals: wide QRS Ischemia: none

What is the rhythm?

There is no discernable sinus activity on this ECG. Hyperkalemia is known to cause loss of P waves, so it is possible sinus conduction is obscured by hyperkalemia; or, the rhythm is junctional or ventricular in origin.

What is the first line treatment?

Membrane stabilizers include calcium and hypertonic saline. Intracellular potassium shifters include insulin/glucose, beta-agonists, and sodium bicarbonate in acidotic patients. Potassium eliminators include loop diuretics and kayexalate. New medications to promote gastrointestinal excretion hold promise (patiromer and sodium zirconium cyclosilicate).[43]

Serum Potassium[43]	Potential ECG Changes	Morphology
5.5-6.5 mEq/L	Tall, peaked T waves with narrow base	
	QT interval shortening	
	ST-segment depression	
6.5-8.0 mEq/L	Peaked T waves	
	PR-interval prolongation	
	P wave decreased amplitude or disappearance	
	QRS widening	
	R-wave amplification	
> 8.0 mEq/L	P-wave absence	
	QRS widening	
	Intraventricular/fascicular/bundle branch blocks	
	Sine wave	

This table shows the expected electrocardiographic changes with given serum potassium levels. It is important to note that potassium-related electrocardiographic changes do not always follow this progression.

Unit 9

Narrow Complex Tachycardia (Regular)
Narrow Complex Tachycardia (Irregular)
Wide Complex Tachycardia

#1 – 90 yo F p/w dyspnea

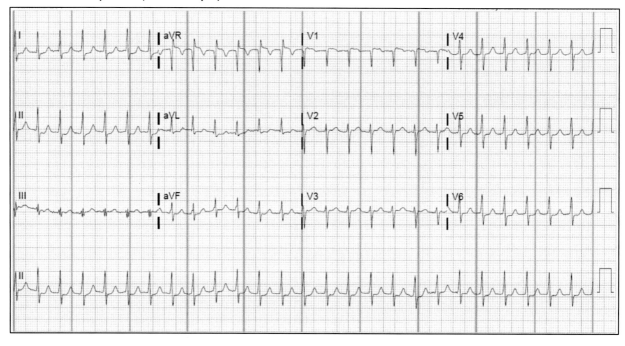

Rate: _____ Rhythm: _____ Axis: _____ Intervals: _____ Ischemia: _____

What is the differential diagnosis for narrow, regular tachycardia with ventricular rate approaching 150?

What ECG features can aid the diagnosis?

What exam findings can aid the diagnosis?

#1 – 90 yo F p/w dyspnea

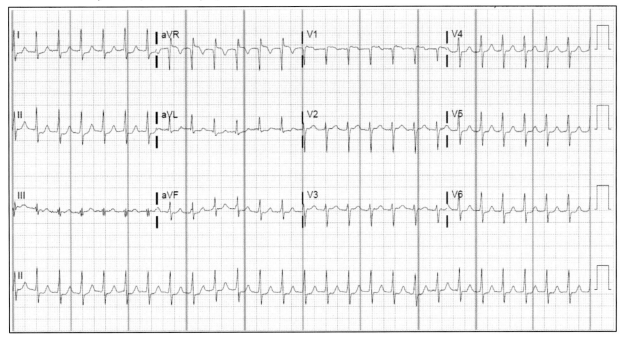

Atrioventricular nodal reentrant tachycardia

Rate: 156 Rhythm: regular Axis: normal Intervals: normal, unable to visualize PR
Ischemia: inferolateral ST depressions and ST elevation in aVR (expected with supraventricular tachycardia)

What is the differential diagnosis for narrow, regular tachycardia with ventricular rate approaching 150?
The differential includes sinus tachycardia, atrioventricular nodal reentrant tachycardia (AVNRT), atrioventricular reentrant tachycardia (AVRT), atrial flutter with 2:1 conduction, and atrial tachycardia.

What ECG features can aid the diagnosis?
In the setting of regular, narrow complex tachycardia, P waves can aid the diagnosis but are often absent. At faster rates, sinus tachycardia can be obscured when P waves are buried within the T waves. P waves in a sawtooth pattern favors atrial flutter (2:1 conduction usually has a ventricular response rate around 150 bpm).[64,68,69] While most cases of AVNRT do not have visible P waves, up to one third of AVNRT cases will show retrograde P' waves immediately following the QRS complex, giving the appearance of a "pseudo-S wave" in the inferior limb leads, or a "pseudo-R wave" in V1. Rarely, atypical "fast-slow" AVNRT can produce retrograde P' waves that immediately precede the QRS complex.[2,68]

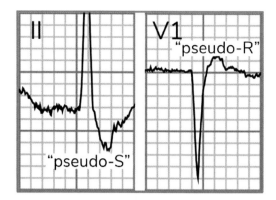

An example of retrograde P waves in a case of AVNRT. The retrograde P waves are labeled as "pseudo-S" in lead II and "pseudo-R" in V1.

What exam findings can aid the diagnosis?

A regular, fixed R-R interval without respiratory variation would oppose the diagnosis of sinus tachycardia, while a labile heart rate that changes with positions or respirations favors sinus tachycardia. While the traditional equation for calculating maximal heart rate (220 – age) has come under scrutiny and other equations exist, it remains a simple bedside tool for helping to determine the likelihood of sinus rhythm.[70] Prominent regular neck pulsations termed "cannon A waves" strongly favor the diagnosis of AVNRT. Cannon A waves are the manifestation of a sudden increase in venous pressure that results from near simultaneous contraction of the atria and ventricles.[35] This patient had obvious "cannon A waves" on exam, lack of R-R variation, and a rate well beyond the expected maximum rate for her age – all supporting the diagnosis of AVNRT. This patient converted to sinus after synchronized electrical cardioversion.

Regular narrow Tachycardia

- Max heart rate (220-age)
- R-R variation
- Flutter waves - consider Lewis Leads
- Retrograde P waves
- Cannon A waves
- Adenosine Challenge

#2 – 76 yo M p/w palpitations

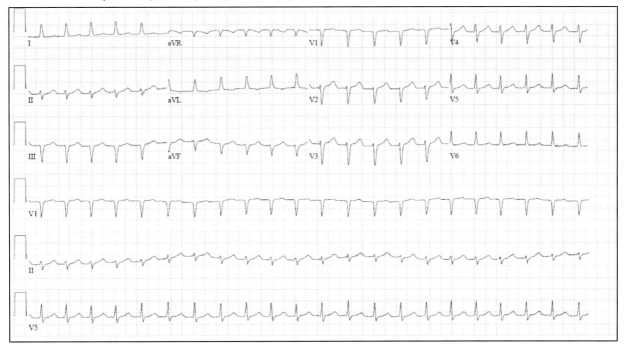

Rate: _____ Rhythm: _____ Axis: _____ Intervals: _____ Ischemia: _____

What diagnostic maneuver can be performed at the bedside to help determine the rhythm?

#2 – 76 yo M p/w palpitations

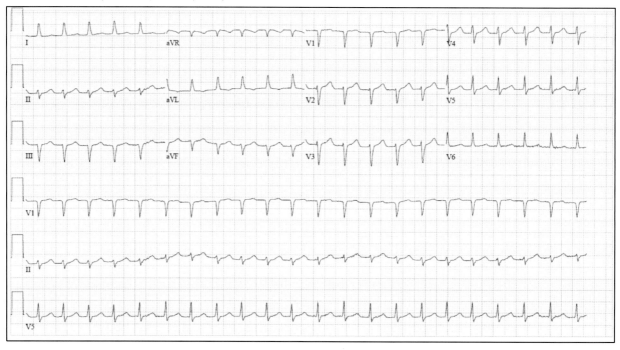

Atrioventricular nodal reentrant tachycardia

Rate: 130 Rhythm: regular Axis: left axis deviation Intervals: normal, unable to visualize PR Ischemia: none

What diagnostic maneuver can be performed at the bedside to help determine the rhythm?

Vagal maneuvers can be attempted at the bedside to help slow the rate to visualize P waves or convert to sinus. Supine repositioning and passive leg raise immediately after a Valsalva strain appear to be more effective than Valsalva alone.[71] Adenosine can be used diagnostically to "unmask" the P waves if present, or therapeutically to convert the patient to a sinus rhythm. This patient converted to sinus rhythm with 12 mg of adenosine. Most textbooks report that the lower rate limit of supraventricular tachycardia is 140 to 150 bpm, but this is not anecdotally true as this case demonstrates.

#3 – 96 yo F p/w fatigue

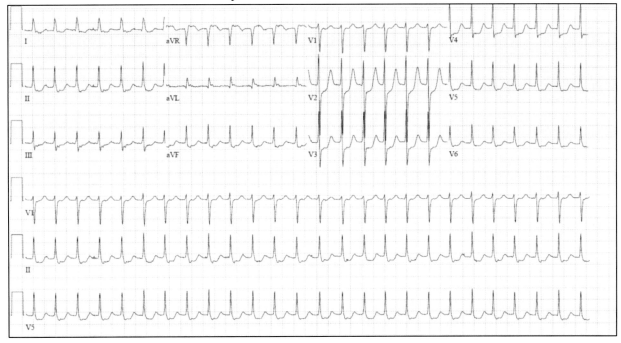

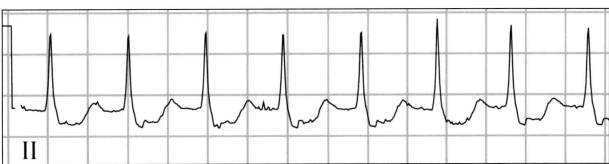

Rate: _____ Rhythm: _____ Axis: _____ Intervals: _____ Ischemia: _____

What is the rhythm?

#3 – 96 yo F p/w fatigue

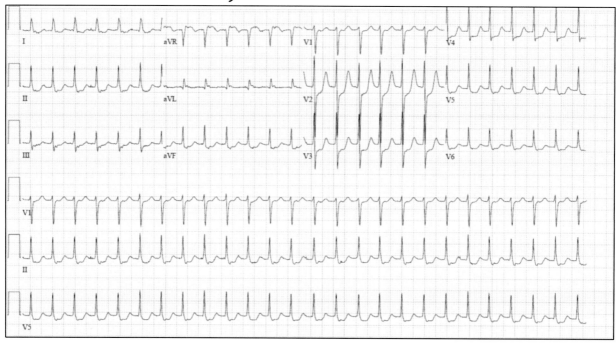

Atrioventricular nodal reentrant tachycardia

Rate: 155 Rhythm: regular Axis: normal Intervals: QTc prolonged but correction formulas not reliable at fast rates, unable to visualize PR Ischemia: diffuse ST depressions with aVR ST

What is the rhythm?

This is another case of atrioventricular nodal reentrant tachycardia. Retrograde P' waves ("pseudo S waves") can be visualized in the inferior leads but resolved after conversion.

Note that the diffuse ST depressions with aVR ST elevation are expected changes of this rhythm and will likely resolve with conversion, as these did.

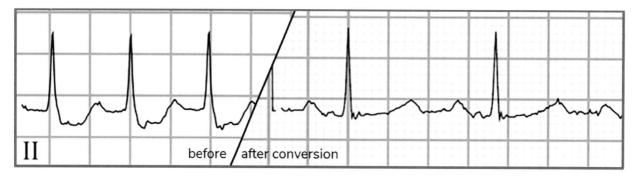

Retrograde P' waves can be seen prior to conversion (left) but are absent after (right).

#4 – 64 yo M p/w dyspnea

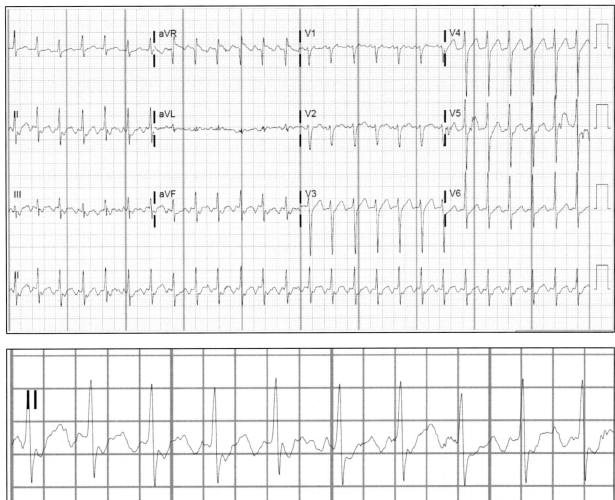

Rate: _____ Rhythm: _____ Axis: _____ Intervals: _____ Ischemia: _____

What are Lewis leads and how might they help?

#4 – 64 yo M p/w dyspnea

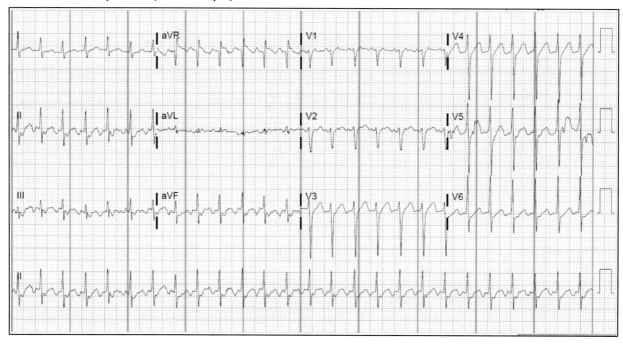

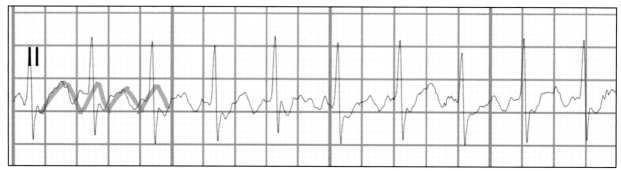

Atrial flutter with 2:1 conduction

Rate: 156 Rhythm: regular Axis: normal Intervals: normal Ischemia: inferolateral ST depressions with aVR ST elevation (expected changes with supraphysiologic rates)

What are Lewis leads and how might they help?

In atrial flutter, the atrial rate can vary from 250 to 400 bpm. Consider 2:1 flutter in any tachycardia with a ventricular rate of 125 to 200 bpm, most commonly close to 150 bpm. Lewis leads can be considered when the diagnosis is in doubt. Lewis leads describe a different positioning of the limb leads in order to better visualize atrial activity.[72]

#4 – 64 yo M p/w dyspnea (after rate control)

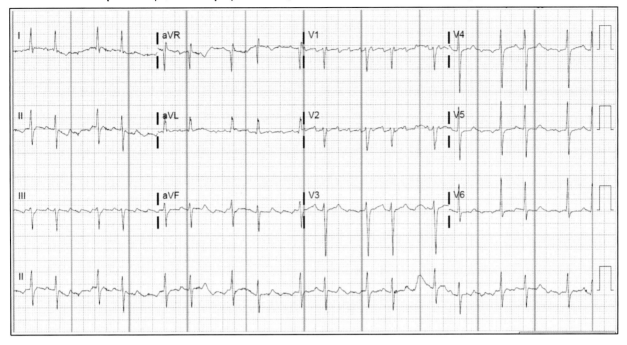

Atrial flutter waves now easily seen (especially in lead III) after rate control with IV metoprolol 5 mg x 3.

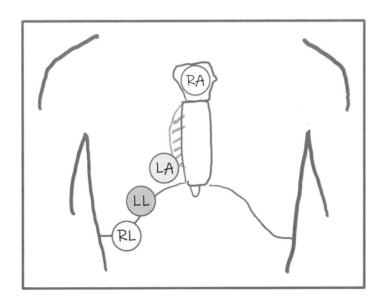

Lewis Leads can help better visualize atrial activity. Lead placement is demonstrated here. RA, right arm electrode; LA, left arm electrode; LL, left lower limb electrode; RL, right lower limb electrode.

#5 – 84 yo M p/w abd pain

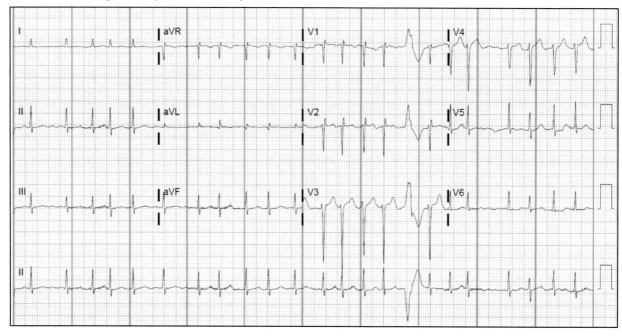

Rate: _____ Rhythm: _____ Axis: _____ Intervals: _____ Ischemia: _____

What's the differential diagnosis for a narrow, irregularly irregular rhythm?

What are the causes of this rhythm?

What's the next step in the management of a stable patient with this rhythm?

What's the next step in the management of an unstable patient with this rhythm?

#5 – 84 yo M p/w abd pain

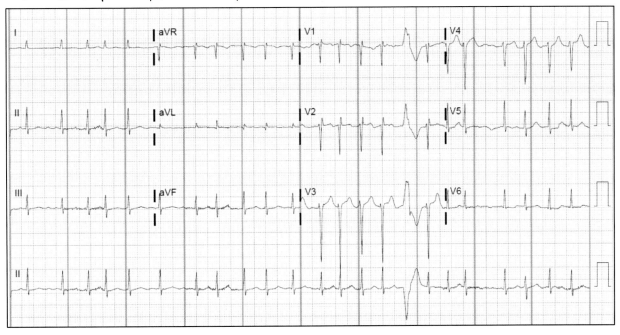

Atrial fibrillation with rapid ventricular response

Rate: 138 Rhythm: irregularly irregular Axis: normal Intervals: normal, unable to visualize P waves Ischemia: none

What's the differential diagnosis for a narrow, irregularly irregular rhythm?

The differential includes atrial fibrillation, multifocal atrial tachycardia, and atrial flutter with variable conduction.

What are the causes of this rhythm?

Any disturbance of atrial architecture (e.g. inflammation, fibrosis, hypertrophy) increases susceptibility. These changes occur most commonly in the setting of heart disease associated with hypertension, coronary artery disease, valvular heart disease, cardiomyopathies, and heart failure (which tend to increase left atrial pressure and alter wall stress). Extracardiac factors that promote atrial fibrillation include sleep apnea, obesity, alcohol/drugs, and hyperthyroidism. "Lone AF" is a historical descriptor that has been variably applied to younger persons without clinical or echocardiographic evidence of cardiopulmonary disease, hypertension, or diabetes mellitus.[73]

What's the next step in the management of a stable patient with this rhythm?

If the duration of onset is reliably less than 48 hours, it is reasonable to offer the patient a rhythm control strategy – either pharmacologic (with amiodarone, dofetilide, flecainide, ibutilide, propafenone, or procainamide) or electrical cardioversion. If the onset is longer than 48 hours, pursue a rate control strategy with either beta blockers or non-dihydropyridine calcium channel blockers as first line agents with a heart rate goal of < 110 bpm. Also, consider anticoagulation after risk stratification with the CHADSVASC score for stroke prevention.[73-75] *Balance w/ HASBLED score*

Always consider secondary causes of atrial fibrillation (i.e. sepsis, pulmonary embolism, etc..) prior to pursuing a rate control strategy as the heart rate could be compensatory.

What's the next step in the management of an unstable patient with this rhythm?
Immediate cardioversion to restore normal atrial activity and ventricular rate.[76] However, special consideration should be given to the acutely ill patient as to whether the heart rate is compensatory. Pathologies that do particularly poorly with faster heart rates and the loss of the "atrial kick" include diastolic dysfunction and mitral stenosis.[77] When considering whether the heart rate is causing adverse effects in the acutely ill patient, esmolol may be the preferred choice owing to its short-acting effects allowing for rapid titration and discontinuation.[78]

#6 – 60 yo M p/w syncope

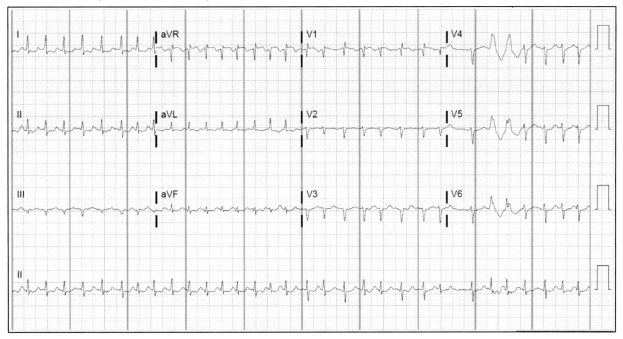

Rate: _____ Rhythm: _____ Axis: _____ Intervals: _____ Ischemia: _____

What is Ashman phenomenon?

Why is it clinically relevant?

#6 – 60 yo M p/w syncope

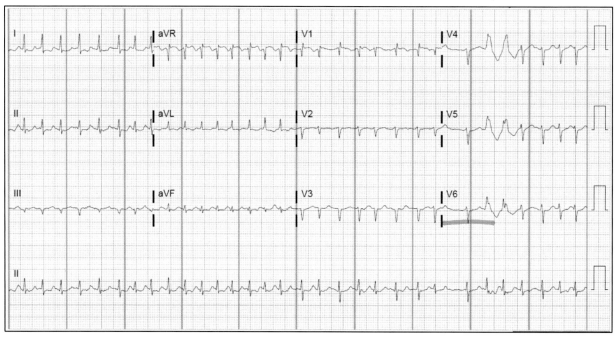

Atrial fibrillation with Ashman phenomenon

Rate: 186 Rhythm: irregularly irregular Axis: normal Intervals: QTc prolonged but correction formulas not reliable at fast rates Ischemia: none

What is Ashman phenomenon?

This is a phenomenon first described in 1947 in which the refractory period of the conduction system is proportional to the length of the preceding cycle, resulting in aberrant conduction when a short cycle is preceded by a longer one. For instance, when a long R-R cycle is followed by a short one, the right bundle is still refractory resulting in an aberrantly conducted complex that has a right bundle branch block morphology. It is commonly mistaken for an ectopic beat. This phenomenon is usually seen in atrial fibrillation.[2]

Why is it clinically relevant?

Several consecutive aberrantly conducted beats can have the appearance of non-sustained ventricular tachycardia when, in fact, they are explained by Ashman phenomenon.

#7 – 58 yo M p/w dyspnea

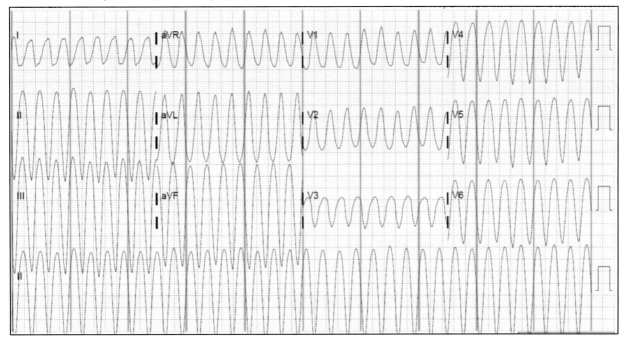

Rate: _____ Rhythm: _____ Axis: _____ Intervals: _____ Ischemia: _____

What's the differential diagnosis for a regular, wide complex tachycardia?

What are the cellular mechanisms for this rhythm?

If stable, what's the next step in management?

If unstable, what's the next step in management?

#7 – 58 yo M p/w dyspnea

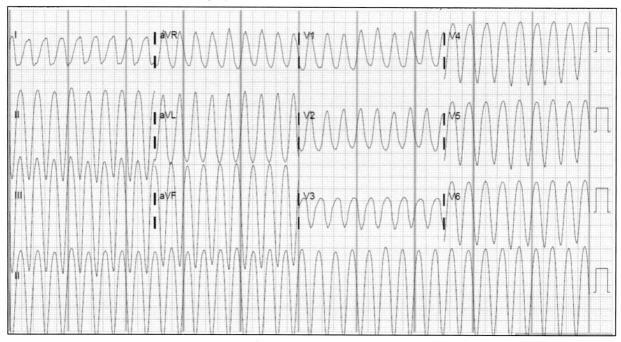

Ventricular tachycardia

Rate: 200 Rhythm: regular Axis: undetermined Intervals: wide QRS Ischemia: n/a

What's the differential diagnosis for a regular, wide complex tachycardia?

The differential includes ventricular tachycardia, supraventricular tachycardia with aberrancy, antidromic atrioventricular tachycardia, and toxicologic/metabolic disturbances (e.g. sodium-channel blockade, hyperkalemia).

What are the cellular mechanisms for this rhythm?

Mechanisms for ventricular arrhythmias include reentry from a prior scar (after a myocardial infarction or a surgically repaired congenital heart disease), triggered activity from early (torsade) or late (digoxin toxicity, catecholaminergic polymorphic ventricular tachycardia, or acute myocardial infarction) after-depolarization, and abnormal automaticity (from acute ischemia or hyperkalemia).[57]

If stable, what's the next step in management?

Pharmacologic cardioversion can be attempted. Procainamide 10 mg/kg over 20 min is likely to be the most effective,[79] but other pharmacologic options exist. Synchronized electrical cardioversion is also safe and effective.

If unstable, what's the next step in management?

Immediate defibrillation.

VT vs SVT with Aberrancy – the CRAM Mnemonic

If any of the following criteria are met, the diagnosis of ventricular tachycardia (VT) should be made; otherwise the patient may be having supraventricular tachycardia (SVT) with aberrancy (i.e. bundle branch block).[80] When in doubt, treat as VT.

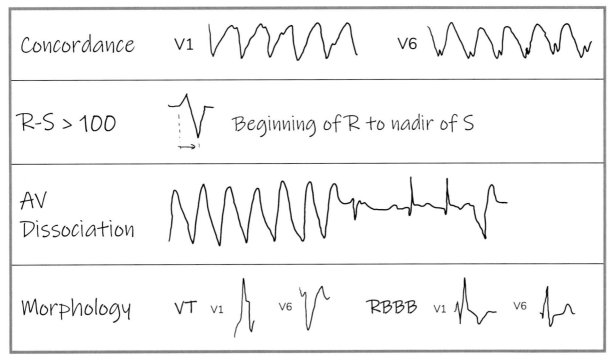

This mnemonic is adapted from the Brugada algorithm, which is one of several algorithms to help differentiate between supraventricular tachycardia with aberrancy and ventricular tachycardia. Concordance describes the situation where QRS complexes are in the same direction (up or down) across the entire precordium (V1 – V6); if this condition is met, ventricular tachycardia is diagnosed. If the beginning of the R wave to the nadir of the S is greater than 100 ms, ventricular tachycardia is diagnosed. If there are signs of AV dissociation (i.e. capture beats, fusion beats, or occasionally P waves can be visualized), ventricular tachycardia is diagnosed. Finally, if the previous three criteria are not met and the morphology suggests aberrancy then ventricular tachycardia is unlikely. Rsr' appearance (as opposed to rsR') in V1 strongly favors ventricular tachycardia. AV, atrioventricular.

It is worth restating that ventricular tachycardia should be the presumed diagnosis for wide complex tachycardia (WCT). Up to 80% of cases of all WCT are ventricular tachycardia, and none of the available algorithms perform well in the acute setting.[81–83] One should be cautious of treating potential VT with AV nodal blockers (as one would for SVT).

#8 – 63 yo M p/w dizziness

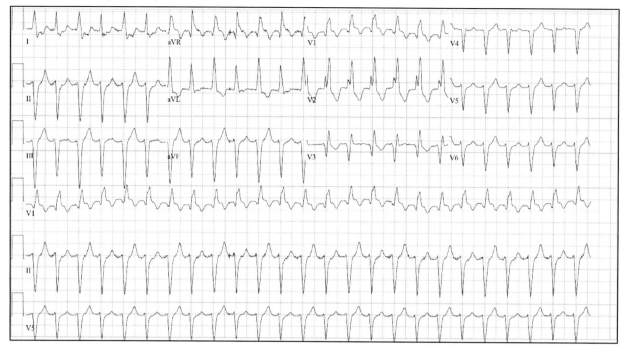

Rate: _____ Rhythm: _____ Axis: _____ Intervals: _____ Ischemia: _____

What is the differential diagnosis for wide complex tachycardia?

What is the rhythm on the presenting ECG?

#8 – 63 yo M p/w dizziness

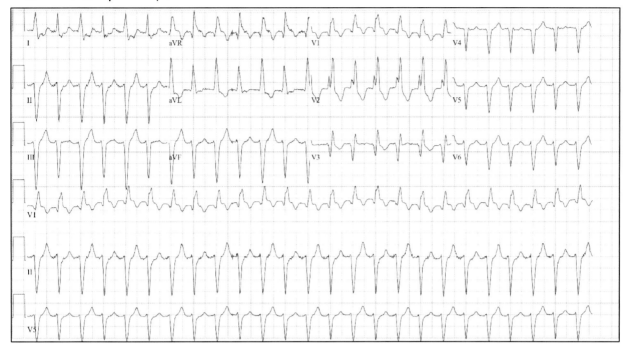

Supraventricular tachycardia with aberrancy

Rate: 150 Rhythm: supraventricular tachycardia Axis: left axis deviation Intervals: wide QRS Ischemia: upsloping lateral ST depressions are expected with supraventricular tachycardia

What is the differential diagnosis for wide complex tachycardia?

The differential includes ventricular tachycardia (VT), supraventricular tachycardia (SVT, e.g. atrial flutter, atrial tachycardia, or atrioventricular nodal reentrant tachycardia) with aberrancy (i.e. bundle branch block), antidromic atrioventricular reentrant tachycardia, and toxicologic/metabolic disturbances (e.g. sodium-channel blockade, hyperkalemia).

What is the rhythm on the presenting ECG?

SVT with aberrancy because the QRS morphology is the exact same as the baseline. There are criteria to help differentiate VT vs SVT with aberrancy,[81] but this is one of the only times SVT with aberrancy can be reliably called – when the baseline ECG shows the same bundle branch block morphology. There are obvious perils of missing VT, and the test characteristics of the various criteria for differentiating VT vs SVT with aberrancy may be insufficient given the serious implications of falsely diagnosing SVT. Therefore, unless there is a compelling alternative (as with this case), VT should be assumed.

#8 – 63 yo M p/w dizziness (baseline ECG)

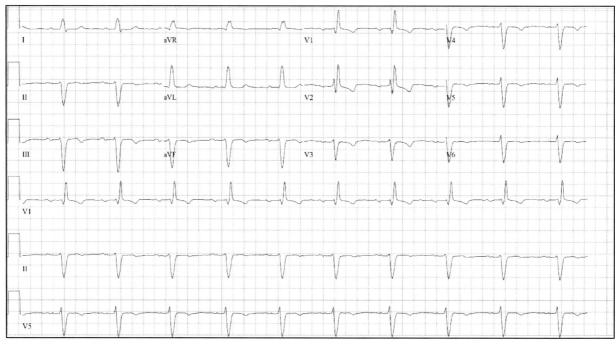

Bifascicular block (RBBB, LAFB)

Rate: 60　Rhythm: sinus　Axis: left axis deviation　Intervals: wide QRS　Ischemia: none

The following is another example of supraventricular tachycardia with aberrancy, this time with a left bundle branch block (LBBB) pattern.

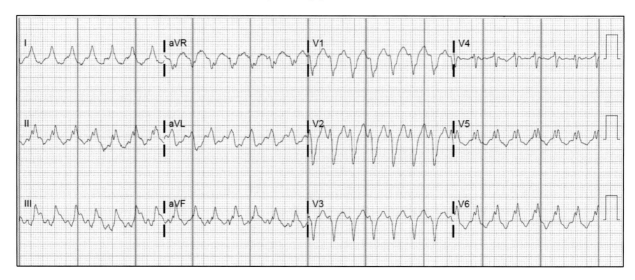

Lack of concordance, R-S < 100 ms, no signs of AV dissociation (e.g. fusion or capture beats), and typical LBBB morphology all make this most likely to be supraventricular tachycardia with aberrancy. In fact, this patient converted with adenosine as expected for atrioventricular nodal reentrant tachycardia.

Unit 10

Paced Rhythms
Pacemaker Malfunction
Sodium Channel Toxicity

#1 – 100 yo F p/w syncope

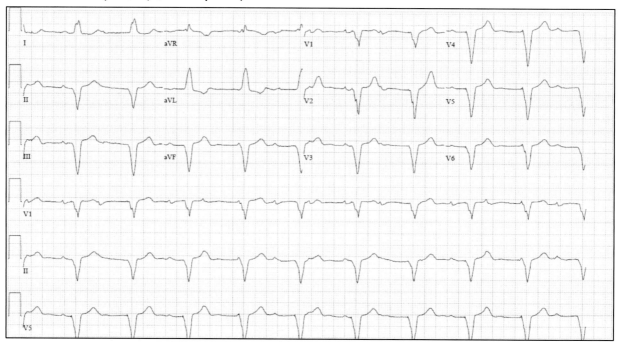

Rate: _____ Rhythm: _____ Axis: _____ Intervals: _____ Ischemia: _____

What is the pacemaker mode?

What are the indications for pacemaker insertion?

#1 – 100 yo F p/w syncope

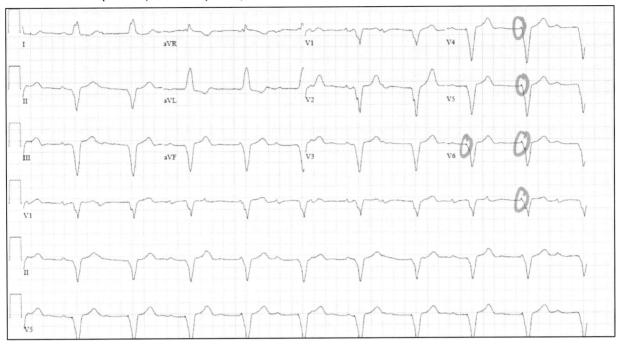

Ventricular paced rhythm

Rate: atrial 100, ventricular 60   Rhythm: ventricular paced   Axis: left axis deviation
Intervals: wide QRS, no PR   Ischemia: none

What is the pacemaker mode?

The mode is likely ventricular sensed, ventricular paced (VVI). Pacemaker spikes can be visualized in V4/5/6. The atrial contractions are ignored. Pacemakers are programmed with five variables, the first three are relevant to emergency physicians and are shown below.[2,84]

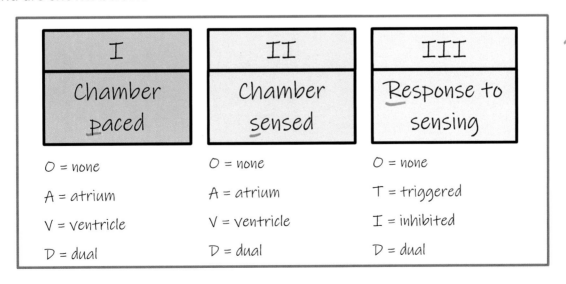

I	II	III
Chamber paced	Chamber sensed	Response to sensing
O = none	O = none	O = none
A = atrium	A = atrium	T = triggered
V = ventricle	V = ventricle	I = inhibited
D = dual	D = dual	D = dual

PSR

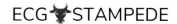

What are the indications for pacemaker insertion?

The following is an incomplete list of indications for pacing (either temporary or permanent as the situation warrants) compiled from the 2018 ACC/AHA/HRS guidelines on the evaluation and management of patients with bradycardia and cardiac conduction delay.[8,85]

1) Sinus node dysfunction (Class I)

2) Second-degree Mobitz II, high-grade, or third-degree atrioventricular block not attributable to reversible causes (Class I)

3) Marked first-degree or second-degree Mobitz type I (Wenckebach) atrioventricular block with symptoms that are clearly attributable to the atrioventricular block (Class IIa)

4) Syncope and bundle branch block with evidence of infranodal disease on electrophysiology testing (Class I)

5) Alternating bundle branch block (Class I)

6) Acute phase of myocardial infarction. Temporary pacing is indicated for refractory or hemodynamically significant bradycardia attributable to sinus node dysfunction or atrioventricular block (Class I). A waiting period is appropriate to determine the need for permanent pacing (Class I).

7) Cardiac resynchronization therapy for severe systolic heart failure (Class I)

8) Neuromuscular disease. Several neuromuscular diseases are associated with atrioventricular block including myotonic muscular dystrophy, Kearns-Sayre syndrome, Erb's dystrophy (limb-girdle), and peroneal muscular atrophy (Class I).

9) Long QT syndrome. High-risk congenital long QT syndromes can be treated with pacemakers to prevent ventricular arrhythmias.

#2 – 76 yo M p/w dyspnea

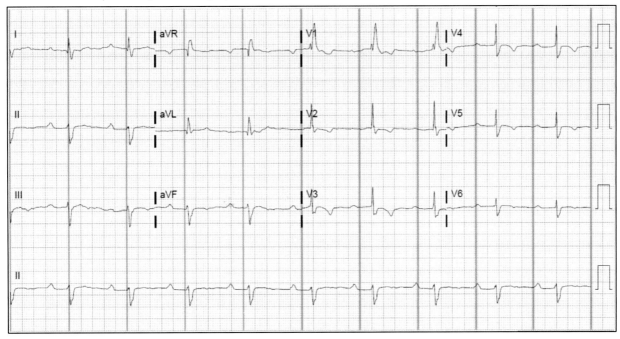

Rate: _____ Rhythm: _____ Axis: _____ Intervals: _____ Ischemia: _____

#2 – 76 yo M p/w dyspnea (subsequent ECG)

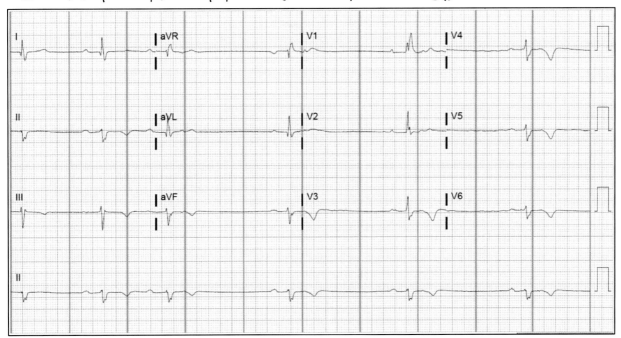

Rate: _____ Rhythm: _____ Axis: _____ Intervals: _____ Ischemia: _____

#2 – 76 yo M p/w dyspnea

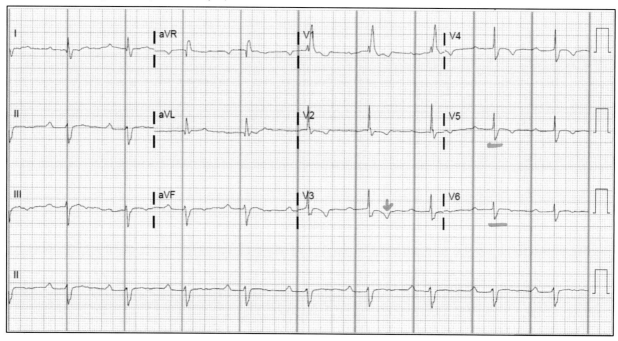

Trifascicular disease

Rate: 60   Rhythm: sinus   Axis: left axis deviation   Intervals: prolonged PR, wide QRS

Ischemia: T wave inversions in V4-6

This patient has trifascicular disease as evidenced by the right bundle branch block, left anterior fascicular block, and first-degree block, which likely represents delayed conduction through the remaining conducting fascicle (see Unit 2, case # 6). The patient subsequently became bradycardic due to sinus node dysfunction (see subsequent ECG). This is a high-risk scenario, given trifascicular disease *and* sinus node dysfunction. This patient clearly needs a permanent pacemaker.

#2 – 76 yo M p/w dyspnea (subsequent ECG)

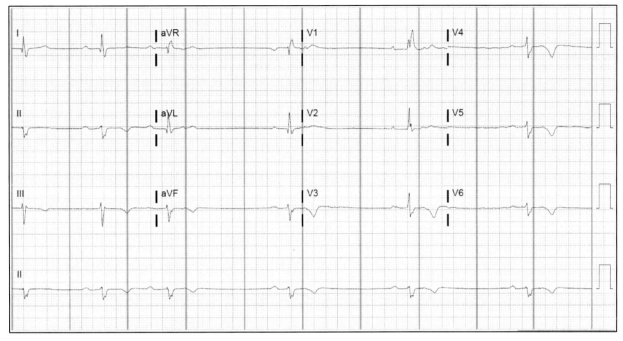

Sinus node dysfunction

Rate: 36 Rhythm: sinus Axis: left axis deviation Intervals: prolonged PR, wide QRS
Ischemia: inferolateral T wave inversions

This patient has trifascicular disease (right bundle branch block, left anterior fascicular block, first-degree atrioventricular block) and sinus node dysfunction with long sinus pauses. Sinus node dysfunction is historically referred to as sick sinus syndrome. It is due to age-related fibrotic degeneration of the sinus node resulting in impaired signal generation and propagation which manifests as sinus pauses, and occasionally episodes of atrial arrhythmias alternating with bradycardia (tachy-brady syndrome).[8] With tachy-brady syndrome, episodes of bradycardia often alternate with atrial fibrillation.

#2 – 76 yo M p/w dyspnea (paced ECG)

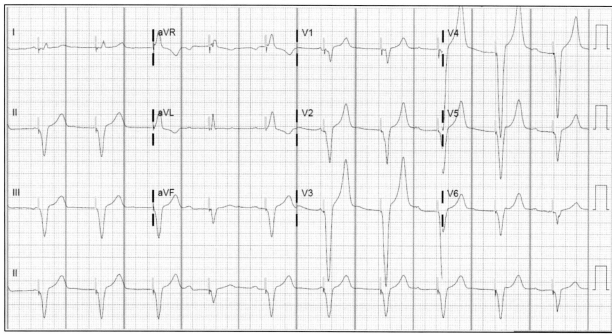

Ventricular paced rhythm

Rate: 60 Rhythm: ventricular paced with atrioventricular dissociation Axis: left axis deviation Intervals: wide QRS, no PR Ischemia: none

The mode is likely VVI, or *demand pacing*, where the presence of an intrinsic depolarization above the pacing rate inhibits pacing. If the intrinsic rate drops below the pacing rate, pacing occurs. This patient has infranodal conduction disease as evidenced by trifascicular disease on the presenting ECG *and* sinus node dysfunction. Neither the sinus node nor the infrahisian conduction system can be trusted to generate a reliable impulse, which is why there are no intrinsic depolarizations evident on this ECG. The most appropriate pacing mode is VVI. VOO or asynchronous is the easiest and most appropriate mode for temporary pacing in the acute setting, but not typically used for permanent pacing.[84]

#3 – 86 yo F p/w cardiac arrest

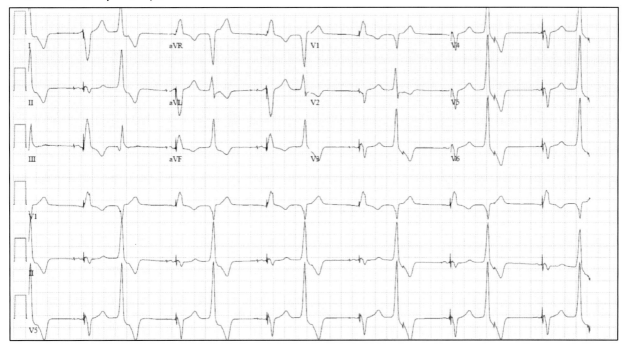

Rate: _____ Rhythm: _____ Axis: _____ Intervals: _____ Ischemia: _____

What is the rhythm?

What bedside maneuver can be done to mitigate this?

#3 – 86 yo F p/w cardiac arrest

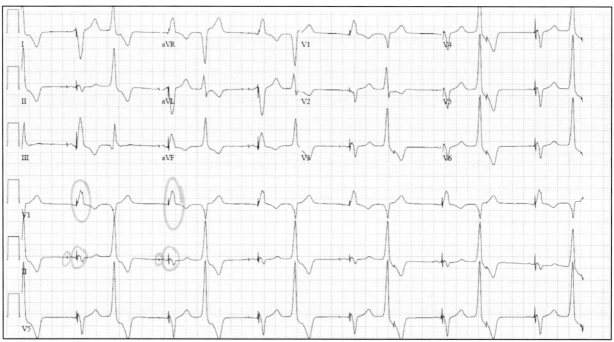

Dual chamber paced with ventricular bigeminy

Rate: 72 <u>Rhythm</u>: dual paced with ventricular bigeminy <u>Axis</u>: paced rhythm with right axis deviation <u>Intervals</u>: wide QRS <u>Ischemia</u>: none

What is the rhythm?

Ventricular bigeminy. Often the second beat of bigeminy is non-perfusing as demonstrated by the image below with an arterial waveform barely registering the bigeminy beat.

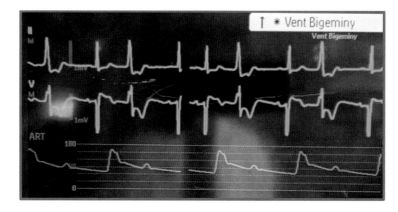

What bedside maneuver can be done to mitigate this?

Practically, this is an over-sensing problem (although it technically is not). The pacemaker is sensing the bigeminy beat and delaying the initiation of the next signal.

Placing a magnet over the pacemaker places it in asynchronous mode, or VOO, a maneuver that may help to mitigate this problem.

Pacemaker Malfunctions

Failure to pace[84,86]

This occurs when the paced stimulus is not generated when expected. Pacemaker spikes are decreased or absent. It is usually caused by oversensing but can also be caused by lead fracture or insulation defect. Oversensing occurs when pacemaker activity is inhibited by inappropriately recognized non-cardiac activity (i.e. skeletal muscle).

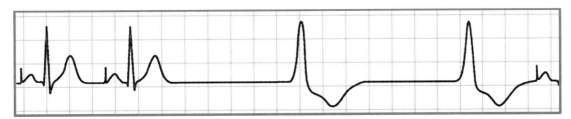

Failure to sense[84,86]

The pacemaker fails to sense native cardiac activity which leads to asynchronous pacing. Pacing spikes can be seen within QRS complexes. This can be caused by a lead insulation break, new intrinsic bundle branch blocks, electrolyte abnormalities, and Class IC antiarrhythmics.

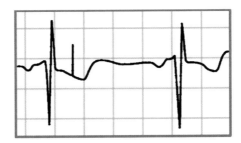

Failure to capture[84,86]

The delivery of a pacing stimulus does not lead to myocardial depolarization. This can be caused by mechanical lead displacement or fracture, electrolyte abnormalities, and ischemia or infarct.

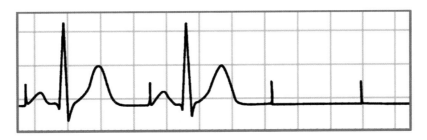

#4 – 51 yo F p/w chest wall spasms

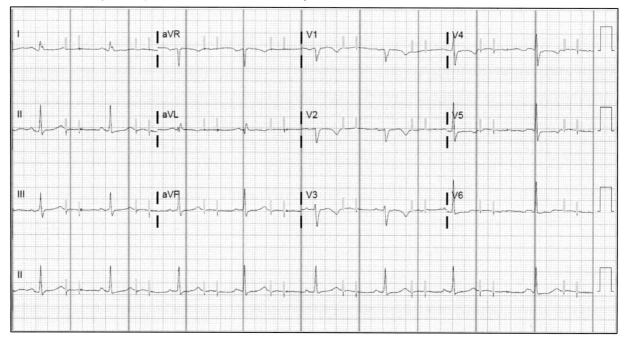

Rate: _____ Rhythm: _____ Axis: _____ Intervals: _____ Ischemia: _____

What type of pacemaker malfunction is this?

#4 – 51 yo F p/w chest wall spasms

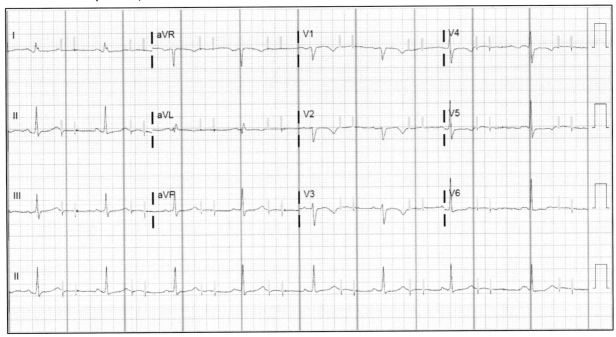

Failure to capture

Rate: 48 Rhythm: sinus bradycardia with intermittent pacer spikes (green lines) Axis: normal Intervals: normal Ischemia: T wave inversions across the precordial leads

What type of pacemaker malfunction is this?

This is failure to capture, which happens when the delivery of a pacing stimulus does not lead to myocardial depolarization. This can be caused by mechanical lead displacement or fracture, electrolyte abnormalities, and ischemia or infarct. In this case, the patient has a dual chamber pacemaker (leads in both right atrium and right ventricle) as evidenced by the couplets of vertical green lines, but the expected atrial and ventricular depolarizations are absent. This was caused by mechanical lead displacement, confirmed on chest x-ray, and is the cause of her chest wall spasms.

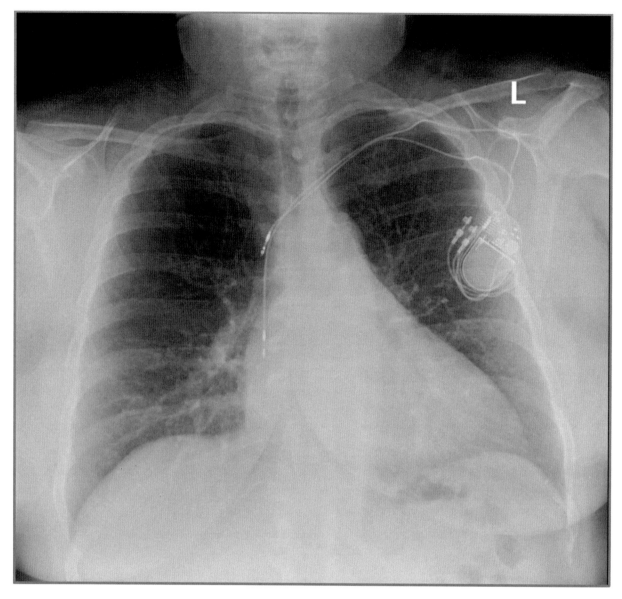

Chest x-ray confirming displaced leads causing failure to capture. The pacemaker leads can be seen wrapped around the pacemaker generator. This represents a rare condition known as Twiddler's syndrome in which the pacemaker malfunctions due to coiling of the device in the skin pocket and resultant lead displacement.[87,88]

#5 – 93 yo M p/w fall

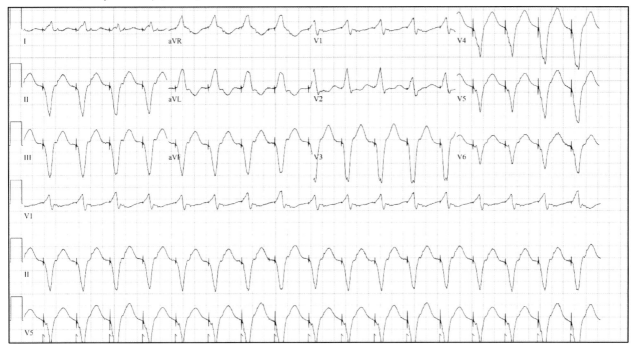

Rate: _____ Rhythm: _____ Axis: _____ Intervals: _____ Ischemia: _____

What is the rhythm?

What are the acute treatment options?

#5 – 93 yo M p/w fall

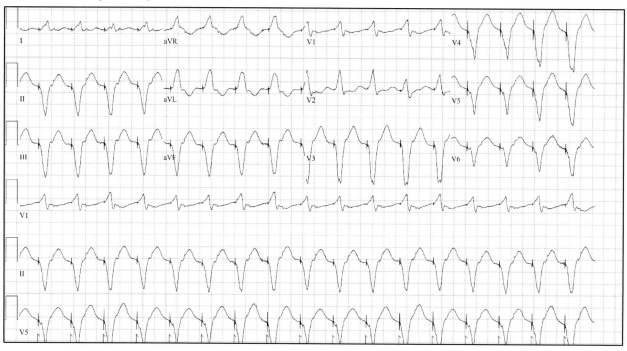

Pacemaker-Mediated Tachycardia

<u>Rate</u>: 105 <u>Rhythm</u>: wide complex tachycardia with pacing spikes <u>Axis</u>: left axis deviation <u>Intervals</u>: wide QRS, prolonged QT <u>Ischemia</u>: anticipated discordant ST changes in setting of ventricular pacing

What is the rhythm?

This is pacemaker-mediated tachycardia (PMT), or endless loop tachycardia. PMT is a reentrant tachycardia in which the pacemaker forms the anterograde pathway and the atrioventricular node forms the retrograde pathway, leading to a pacemaker-sensed retrograde P' wave. It typically occurs in patients with dual chamber pacemakers in DDD mode. The rate is usually at or near the programmed upper limit.[89–91]

What are the acute treatment options?

PMT can be terminated by slowing conduction through the atrioventricular node (e.g. adenosine) or activating asynchronous mode by placing a magnet over the pacing generator. Most pacemakers have programmed algorithms to prevent PMT from happening.[89]

#6 – 45 yo M status post unknown ingestion

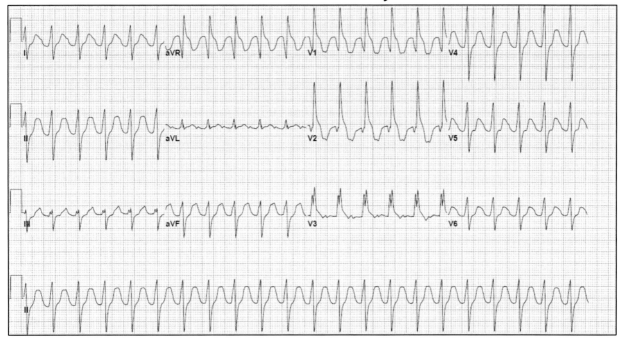

Rate: _____ Rhythm: _____ Axis: _____ Intervals: _____ Ischemia: _____

What was the likely ingestion?

What ECG features suggest the diagnosis?

What is the next step in management?

#6 – 45 yo M status post unknown ingestion

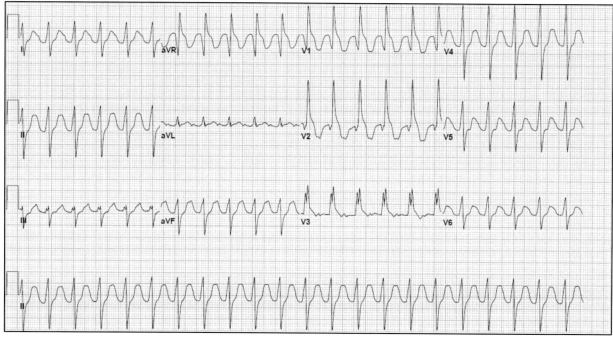

Sodium channel toxicity

<u>Rate</u>: 132 <u>Rhythm</u>: sinus <u>Axis</u>: indeterminate <u>Intervals</u>: wide QRS, prolonged QT
<u>Ischemia</u>: none

What was the likely ingestion?

The likely ingestion is a sodium channel blocking drug. Classily, sodium channel toxicity was described in tricyclic overdoses,[92] but many drugs can cause toxic sodium channel effects including antiarrhythmics (lidocaine, phenytoin, propafenone, flecainide, amiodarone, sotalol), antiepileptic medications (carbamazepine, lamotrigine), selective serotonin reuptake inhibitors (citalopram, fluoxetine), antihistamines (diphenhydramine), propranolol, cyclobenzaprine, and others.[93]

What ECG features suggest the diagnosis?

Widened QRS, prolonged QT, right axis deviation, tall terminal R in aVR.

What is the next step in management?

Patients with sodium channel toxicity need a sodium load. One of the most effective ways of delivering sodium is via 8.4% sodium bicarbonate, which has the dual effect of loading with extracellular sodium and alkalinizing the serum pH, favoring the neutral (ie, non-ionized) form of the drug and making it less available to bind to sodium channels.[94] Give 1-2 ampules of 8.4% sodium bicarbonate and repeat the

ECG, continue until the QRS is < 100 ms to reduce the risk of seizures and arrythmias.[92,93]

#6 – After 8.4% sodium bicarbonate

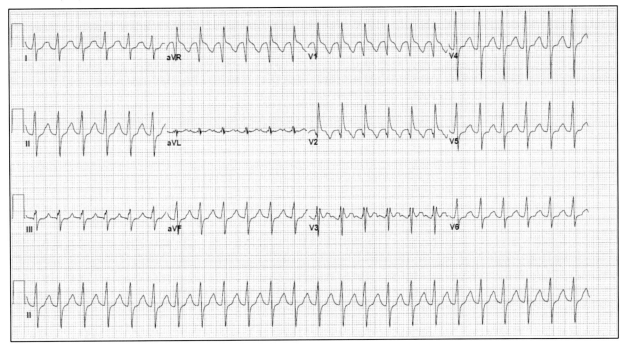

#6 – After more 8.4% sodium bicarbonate

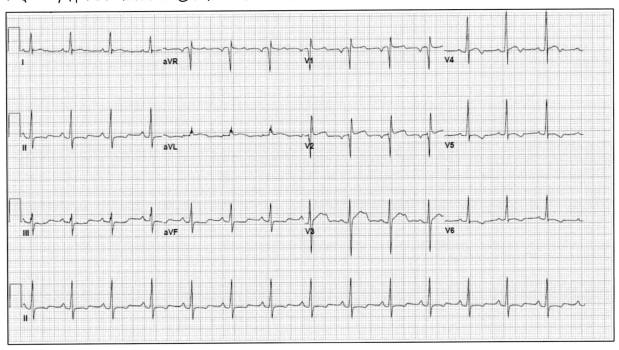

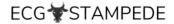

References

1. O'gara P, Kushner F, Aschei D, et al. 2013 ACCF/AHA Guideline for the Management of ST-Elevation Myocardial Infarction. *Circulation*. 2013;127(4):e362-425. doi:10.1161/CIR.0b013e3182742cf6

2. Wagner GS, Strauss DG. *Marriott's Practical Electrocardiography*. 12th ed. Philadelphia, PA: Lippincott Williams & Wilkins; 2014.

3. Zimetbaum PJ, Josephson ME. Use of the electrocardiogram in acute myocardial infarction. *N Engl J Med*. 2003;348(10):933-940. doi:10.1056/NEJMra022700

4. Elizari M V., Acunzo RS, Ferreiro M. Hemiblocks revisited. *Circulation*. 2007;115(9):1154-1163. doi:10.1161/CIRCULATIONAHA.106.637389

5. Rosenbaum MB, Elizari M V., Lazzari JO, Nau GJ, Levi RJ, Halpern MS. Intraventricular trifascicular blocks. Review of the literature and classification. *Am Heart J*. 1969;78(4):450-459. doi:10.1016/0002-8703(69)90478-5

6. Rosenbaum MB. The hemiblocks: diagnostic criteria and clinical significance. *Mod Concepts Cardiovasc Dis*. 1970;39(12):141-146. http://www.ncbi.nlm.nih.gov/pubmed/5497472. Accessed March 2, 2020.

7. Surawicz B, Childers R, Deal BJ, Gettes LS. AHA/ACCF/HRS Recommendations for the Standardization and Interpretation of the Electrocardiogram. Part III: Intraventricular Conduction Disturbances A Scientific Statement From the American Heart Association Electrocardiography and Arrhythmias Committee, Council on Clinical Cardiology; the American College of Cardiology Foundation; and the Heart Rhythm Society. *J Am Coll Cardiol*. 2009. doi:10.1016/j.jacc.2008.12.013

8. Kusumoto FM, Schoenfeld MH, Barrett C, et al. 2018 ACC/AHA/HRS Guideline on the Evaluation and Management of Patients With Bradycardia and Cardiac Conduction Delay: A Report of the American College of Cardiology/American Heart Association Task Force on Clinical Practice Guidelines and the Heart Rhyth. *Circulation*. 2019;140(8):e382-e482. doi:10.1161/CIR.0000000000000628

9. Costa D Da, Brady WJ, Edhouse J. Bradycardias and Atrioventricular conduction block. *Br Med J*. 2002;324(March):535-538. doi:10.1136/bmj.324.7336.535

10. Sgarbossa EB, Investigators G-1. Electrocardiographic Diagnosis of Evolving Acute Myocardial Infarction in the Presence of Left Bundle-Branch Block. *N Engl J Med*. 1996;334(8):481-487. doi:10.1021/ja00009a021

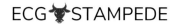
11. Meyers HP, Limkakeng AT, Jaffa EJ, et al. Validation of the modified Sgarbossa criteria for acute coronary occlusion in the setting of left bundle branch block: A retrospective case-control study. *Am Heart J.* 2015;170(6):1255-1264. doi:10.1016/j.ahj.2015.09.005

12. Ibanez B, James S, Agewall S, et al. 2017 ESC Guidelines for the management of acute myocardial infarction in patients presenting with ST-segment elevation. *Eur Heart J.* 2018;39(2):119-177. doi:10.1093/eurheartj/ehx393

13. Di Marco A, Rodriguez M, Cinca J, et al. New Electrocardiographic Algorithm for the Diagnosis of Acute Myocardial Infarction in Patients With Left Bundle Branch Block. *J Am Heart Assoc.* 2020;9(14). doi:10.1161/JAHA.119.015573

14. Moore EN, Spear JF, Boineau JP. Recent Electrophysiologic Studies on the Wolff-Parkinson-White Syndrome. *N Engl J Med.* 1973;289(18):956-963. doi:10.1056/nejm197311012891808

15. Benson DW, Cohen MI. Wolff-Parkinson-White syndrome: Lessons learnt and lessons remaining. *Cardiol Young.* 2017;27(S1):S62-S67. doi:10.1017/S1047951116002250

16. Ayer A, Terkelsen CJ. Difficult ECGs in STEMI: Lessons learned from serial sampling of pre- and in-hospital ECGs. *J Electrocardiol.* 2014;47(4):448-458. doi:10.1016/j.jelectrocard.2014.03.010

17. Waldo SW, Brenner DA, Li S, Alexander K, Ganz P. Reperfusion times and in-hospital outcomes among patients with an isolated posterior myocardial infarction: Insights from the National Cardiovascular Data Registry (NCDR). *Am Heart J.* 2014;167(3):350-354. doi:10.1016/j.ahj.2013.11.011

18. Meyers HP, Dodd KW, Smith SW. Dr. Smith's ECG Blog: Barcelona Rule on Left Bundle Branch Block: Lots of Issues. Dr. Smith's ECG Blog. http://hqmeded-ecg.blogspot.com/2020/11/barcelona-rule-on-left-bundle-branch.html. Published 2020. Accessed January 2, 2021.

19. de Pádua F, Pereirinha A, Marques N, Lopes MG, Macfarlane PW. Conduction Defects. In: Macfarlane PW, van Oosterom A, Pahlm O, Kligfield P, Janse M, Camm J, eds. *Comprehensive Electrocardiology.* London: Springer London; 2010:547-604. doi:10.1007/978-1-84882-046-3_14

20. Xiong Y, Wang L, Liu W, Hankey GJ, Xu B, Wang S. The Prognostic Significance of Right Bundle Branch Block: A Meta-analysis of Prospective Cohort Studies. *Clin Cardiol.* 2015;38(10):604-613. doi:10.1002/clc.22454

21. Widimsky P, Roháč F, Štásek J, et al. Primary angioplasty in acute myocardial infarction with right bundle branch block: Should new onset right bundle branch block be added to future guidelines as an indication for reperfusion therapy? *Eur Heart J.* 2012;33(1):86-95. doi:10.1093/eurheartj/ehr291

22. Ginzton LE, Laks MM. The differential diagnosis of acute pericarditis from the normal variant: New electrocardiographic criteria. *Circulation.* 1982;65(5):1004-1009. doi:10.1161/01.CIR.65.5.1004

23. Haïssaguerre M, Derval N, Sacher F, et al. Sudden Cardiac Arrest Associated with Early Repolarization. *N Engl J Med.* 2008;358(19):2016-2023. doi:10.1056/NEJMoa071968

24. Cooper BL, Fisher KM, Chathampally Y. Man With Left-Sided Chest Pain. *Ann Emerg Med.* 2018;72(5):558-561. doi:10.1016/j.annemergmed.2017.09.006

25. Engel J, Brady WJ, Mattu A, Perron AD. Electrocardiographic ST segment elevation: Left ventricular aneurysm. *Am J Emerg Med.* 2002;20(3):238-242. doi:10.1053/ajem.2002.32634

26. Klein LR, Shroff GR, Beeman W, Smith SW. Electrocardiographic criteria to differentiate acute anterior ST-elevation myocardial infarction from left ventricular aneurysm. *Am J Emerg Med.* 2015;33(6):786-790. doi:10.1016/j.ajem.2015.03.044

27. Mills RM, Young E, Gorlin R, Lesch M. Natural history of S-T segment elevation after acute myocardial infarction. *Am J Cardiol.* 1975;35(5):609-614. doi:10.1016/0002-9149(75)90045-4

28. Meizlish JL, Berger HJ, Plankey M, Errico D, Levy W, Zaret BL. Functional Left Ventricular Aneurysm Formation after Acute Anterior Transmural Myocardial Infarction. *N Engl J Med.* 1984;311(16):1001-1006. doi:10.1056/nejm198410183111601

29. Kosuge M, Ebina T, Hibi K, et al. An early and simple predictor of severe left main and/or three-vessel disease in patients with nonst-segment elevation acute coronary syndrome. *Am J Cardiol.* 2011;107(4):495-500. doi:10.1016/j.amjcard.2010.10.005

30. Knotts RJ, Wilson JM, Kim E, Huang HD, Birnbaum Y. Diffuse ST depression with ST elevation in aVR: Is this pattern specific for global ischemia due to left main coronary artery disease? *J Electrocardiol.* 2013;46(3):240-248. doi:10.1016/j.jelectrocard.2012.12.016

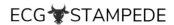

31. Witkov RB, Cooper BL. An Ominous ECG Pattern. *Ann Emerg Med.* 2019;73(4):406-408. doi:10.1016/j.annemergmed.2018.04.024

32. Miranda D, Lobo A, Walsh B. New insights into the use of the 12-lead electrocardiogram for diagnosing acute myocardial infarction in the emergency department. *Can J Cardiol.* 2018;34:132-145.

33. Kukla P, Macintyre W, Fijorek K. Electrocardiographic abnonmralities in patients with acute pulmonary emoblism complicated by cardiogenic shock. *Am J Emerg Med.* 2014;32:507-510.

34. Wagner GS, Macfarlane P, Wellens H, et al. AHA/ACCF/HRS Recommendations for the Standardization and Interpretation of the Electrocardiogram. Part V: Electrocardiogram Changes Associated With Cardiac Chamber Hypertrophy. *Circulation.* 2009;53(11):1003-1011. doi:10.1016/j.jacc.2008.12.016

35. Cooper BL, Beyene JA. Atrioventricular nodal reentrant tachycardia and cannon A waves: A case report. *Am J Emerg Med.* 2018. doi:10.1016/j.ajem.2018.11.016

36. Mani BC, Pavri BB. Dual atrioventricular nodal pathways physiology: A review of relevant anatomy, electrophysiology, and electrocardiographic manifestations. *Indian Pacing Electrophysiol J.* 2014;14(1):12-25. doi:10.1016/S0972-6292(16)30711-2

37. Thygesen K, Alpert JS, Jaffe AS, et al. *Fourth Universal Definition of Myocardial Infarction (2018).*; 2018. doi:10.1016/j.gheart.2018.08.004

38. Macias M, Peachey J, Mattu A, Brady WJ. The electrocardiogram in the ACS patient: High-risk electrocardiographic presentations lacking anatomically oriented ST-segment elevation. *Am J Emerg Med.* 2016;34(3):611-617. doi:10.1016/j.ajem.2015.11.047

39. LeWinter MM. Acute Pericarditis. *N Engl J Med.* 2017;371(25):349-359. doi:10.1016/j.pcad.2016.12.001

40. Witting MD, Hu KM, Westreich AA, Tewelde S, Farzad A, Mattu A. Evaluation of Spodick's Sign and Other Electrocardiographic Findings as Indicators of STEMI and Pericarditis. *J Emerg Med.* March 2020. doi:10.1016/j.jemermed.2020.01.017

41. Spodick DH. Electrocardiogram in acute pericarditis. Distributions of morphologic and axial changes by stages. *Am J Cardiol.* 1974;33(4):470-474. doi:10.1016/0002-9149(74)90603-1

42. Imazio M, Brucato A, Cemin R, et al. A Randomized Trial of Colchicine for Acute Pericarditis. *N Engl J Med.* 2013;369(16):1522-1528.

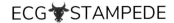
doi:10.1056/NEJMoa1208536

43. Long B, Warix JR, Koyfman A. Controversies in Management of Hyperkalemia. *J Emerg Med.* 2018;55(2):192-205. doi:10.1016/j.jemermed.2018.04.004

44. Durfey N, Lehnhof B, Bergeson A, et al. Severe Hyperkalemia: Can the Electrocardiogram Risk Stratify for Short-term Adverse Events? *West J Emerg Med.* 2017;18(5):963-971. doi:10.5811/westjem.2017.6.33033

45. Diercks DB, Shumaik GM, Harrigan RA, Brady WJ, Chan TC. Electrocardiographic manifestations: Electrolyte abnormalities. *J Emerg Med.* 2004;27(2):153-160. doi:10.1016/j.jemermed.2004.04.006

46. Dezman ZD, Mattu A, Body R. Utility of the History and Physical Examination in the Detection of Acute Coronary Syndromes in Emergency Department Patients. *West J Emerg Med.* 2017;18(4):752-760. doi:10.5811/westjem.2017.3.32666

47. Body R, Carley S, Wibberley C, McDowell G, Ferguson J, Mackway-Jones K. The value of symptoms and signs in the emergent diagnosis of acute coronary syndromes. *Resuscitation.* 2010;81(3):281-286. doi:10.1016/j.resuscitation.2009.11.014

48. Moye S, Carney MF, Holstege C, Mattu A, Brady WJ. The electrocardiogram in right ventricular myocardial infarction. *Am J Emerg Med.* 2005;23(6):793-799. doi:10.1016/j.ajem.2005.04.001

49. de Winter RJ, Verouden NJW, Wellens HJJ, Wilde AAM. A New ECG Sign of Proximal LAD Occlusion. *N Engl J Med.* 2008;359(19):2071-2073. doi:10.1056/NEJMc0804737

50. Goebel M, Bledsoe J, Orford JL, Mattu A, Brady WJ. A new ST-segment elevation myocardial infarction equivalent pattern? Prominent T wave and J-point depression in the precordial leads associated with ST-segment elevation in lead aVr. *Am J Emerg Med.* 2014;32(3):287.e5-287.e8. doi:10.1016/j.ajem.2013.09.037

51. Sieira J, Brugada P. The definition of the Brugada syndrome. *Eur Heart J.* 2017;38(40):3029-3034. doi:10.1093/eurheartj/ehx490

52. de Luna A, Garcia-Niebla J, Baranchuk A. New Electrocardiographic Features in Brugada Syndrome. *Curr Cardiol Rev.* 2014;10(3):175-180. doi:10.2174/1573403x10666140514101546

53. Sharifi M, Bay C, Skrocki L, Rahimi F, Mehdipour M. Moderate pulmonary embolism treated with thrombolysis (from the "mOPETT" Trial). *Am J Cardiol.*

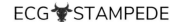

2013;111(2):273-277. doi:10.1016/j.amjcard.2012.09.027

54. Kline JA, Nordenholz KE, Courtney DM, et al. Treatment of submassive pulmonary embolism with tenecteplase or placebo: Cardiopulmonary outcomes at 3 months: Multicenter double-blind, placebo-controlled randomized trial. *J Thromb Haemost*. 2014;12(4):459-468. doi:10.1111/jth.12521

55. Meyer G, Vicaut E, Danays T, et al. Fibrinolysis for Patients with Intermediate-Risk Pulmonary Embolism. *N Engl J Med*. 2014;370(15):1402-1411. doi:10.1056/NEJMoa1302097

56. Sharifi M, Vajo Z, Javadpoor S, et al. Pulseless electrical activity in pulmonary embolism treated with thrombolysis (from the "PEAPETT" study). *Am J Emerg Med*. 2016;34(10):1963-1967. doi:10.1016/j.ajem.2016.06.094

57. Al-Khatib SM, Stevenson WG, Ackerman MJ, et al. 2017 AHA/ACC/HRS Guideline for Management of Patients With Ventricular Arrhythmias and the Prevention of Sudden Cardiac Death. *J Am Coll Cardiol*. 2018;72(14):e91-e220. doi:10.1161/CIR.0000000000000549

58. Isbister GK. Risk assessment of drug-induced QT prolongation. *Aust Prescr*. 2015;38(1):20-24. doi:10.18773/austprescr.2015.003

59. Rischall ML, Smith SW, Friedman AB. Screening for QT Prolongation in the Emergency Department: Is There a Better "Rule of Thumb?" *West J Emerg Med*. 2020;226(2). doi:10.5811/westjem.2019.10.40381

60. Danzi S, Klein I. Thyroid disease and the cardiovascular system. *Endocrinol Metab Clin North Am*. 2014;43(2):517-528. doi:10.1016/j.ecl.2014.02.005

61. Doshi HH, Giudici MC. The EKG in hypothermia and hyperthermia. *J Electrocardiol*. 2015;48(2):203-209. doi:10.1016/j.jelectrocard.2014.12.001

62. Burch GE, Meyes R, Abildskov JA. A new electrocardiographic pattern observed in cerebrovascular accidents. *Circulation*. 1954;9(5):719-723. doi:10.1161/01.CIR.9.5.719

63. Stone J, Mor-Avi V, Ardelt A, Lang RM. Frequency of Inverted Electrocardiographic T Waves (Cerebral T Waves) in Patients With Acute Strokes and Their Relation to Left Ventricular Wall Motion Abnormalities. *Am J Cardiol*. 2018;121(1):120-124. doi:10.1016/j.amjcard.2017.09.025

64. Link MS. Evaluation and Initial Treatment of Supraventricular Tachycardia. *N Engl J Med*. 2012;367(15):1438-1448. doi:10.1056/NEJMcp1111259

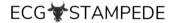

65. Gersh BJ, Maron BJ, Bonow RO, et al. 2011 ACCF/AHA guideline for the diagnosis and treatment of hypertrophic cardiomyopathy: A report of the American College of Cardiology Foundation/American Heart Association Task Force on Practice Guidelines Developed in Collaboration with the American Ass. *J Am Coll Cardiol.* 2011;58(25):e212-e260. doi:10.1016/j.jacc.2011.06.011

66. Zwaan D, Biir FWHM, Wellens HJJ. Characteristic electrocardiogric pattern indicating a critical stenosis high in left anteior descending coronary artery in patients admitted because of impending myocardial infarction. *Am Hear J.* 1982;103(4):730-736.

67. Madias JE. Low QRS voltage and its causes. *J Electrocardiol.* 2008;41(6):498-500. doi:10.1016/j.jelectrocard.2008.06.021

68. Katritsis DG, Camm AJ. Atrioventricular nodal reentrant tachycardia. *Circulation.* 2010;122(8):831-840. doi:10.1161/CIRCULATIONAHA.110.936591

69. Whinnett ZI, Sohaib SMA, Davies DW. Diagnosis and management of supraventricular tachycardia. *Bmj.* 2012;345(dec11 1):e7769-e7769. doi:10.1136/bmj.e7769

70. Kitzman DW. Chronotropic incompetence: Causes, implications, and management. *Circulation.* 2011;123(9):1010-1020. doi:10.1161/CIRCULATIONAHA.110.940577

71. Appelboam A, Reuben A, Mann C, et al. Postural modifi cation to the standard Valsalva manoeuvre for emergency treatment of supraventricular tachycardias (REVERT): a randomised controlled trial. :1747-1753. doi:10.1016/S0140-6736(15)61485-4

72. Bakker ALM, Nijkerk G, Groenemeijer BE, et al. The lewis lead: Making recognition of p waves easy during wide QRS complex tachycardia. *Circulation.* 2009;119(24). doi:10.1161/CIRCULATIONAHA.109.852053

73. January CT, Wann LS, Alpert JS, et al. AHA / ACC / HRS Practice Guideline 2014 AHA / ACC / HRS Guideline for the Management of Patients With Atrial Fibrillation A Report of the American College of Cardiology / American Heart Association Task Force on Practice Guidelines and the Heart Rhythm So. *Circulation.* 2014;130(23):199-267. doi:10.1161/CIR.0000000000000041

74. Van Gelder IC, Groenveld H, Crijns H, et al. Lenient versus Strict Rate Control in Patients with Atrial Fibrillation. *N Engl J Med.* 2010;362(15):1363-1373.

75. Stiell IG, Clement CM, Perry JJ, et al. EM Advances Association of the Ottawa

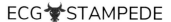
Aggressive Protocol with rapid discharge of emergency department patients with recent-onset atrial fibrillation or flutter. 2010;12(3):181-191.

76. January CT, Wann LS, Alpert JS, et al. 2014 AHA/ACC/HRS guideline for the management of patients with atrial fibrillation: A report of the American College of cardiology/American heart association task force on practice guidelines and the heart rhythm society. *Circulation.* 2014;130(23):e199-e267. doi:10.1161/CIR.0000000000000041

77. Bosch NA, Cimini J, Walkey AJ. Atrial Fibrillation in the ICU. *Chest.* 2018;154(6):1424-1434. doi:10.1016/j.chest.2018.03.040

78. Abrams J, Allen J, Allin D, et al. Efficacy and safety of esmolol vs propranolol in the treatment of supraventricular tachyarrhythmias: A multicenter double-blind clinical trial. *Am Heart J.* 1985;110(5):913-922. doi:10.1016/0002-8703(85)90185-1

79. Ortiz M, Martin A, Arribas F, et al. Randomized comparison of intravenous procainamide vs. intravenous amiodarone for the acute treatment of tolerated wide QRS tachycardia: The PROCAMIO study. *Eur Heart J.* 2017;38(17):1329-1335. doi:10.1093/eurheartj/ehw230

80. Brugada P, Brugada J, Mont L, Smeets J, Andries EW. A New Approach to the Differential Diagnosis of a Regular Tachycardia With a Wide QRS Complex. *Circulation.* 1991;83:1649-1659.

81. Vereckei A. Current Algorithms for the Diagnosis of wide QRS Complex Tachycardias. *Curr Cardiol Rev.* 2014;10(3):262-276. doi:10.2174/1573403x10666140514103309

82. Baxi RP, Hart KW, Vereckei A, et al. Vereckei criteria as a diagnostic tool amongst emergency medicine residents to distinguish between ventricular tachycardia and supra-ventricular tachycardia with aberrancy. *J Cardiol.* 2012;59(3):307-312. doi:10.1016/j.jjcc.2011.11.007

83. Szelényi Z, Duray G, Katona G, et al. Comparison of the "real-life" diagnostic value of two recently published electrocardiogram methods for the differential diagnosis of wide QRS complex tachycardias. *Acad Emerg Med.* 2013;20(11):1121-1130. doi:10.1111/acem.12247

84. Mulpuru SK, Madhavan M, McLeod CJ, Cha YM, Friedman PA. Cardiac Pacemakers: Function, Troubleshooting, and Management: Part 1 of a 2-Part Series. *J Am Coll Cardiol.* 2017;69(2):189-210. doi:10.1016/j.jacc.2016.10.061

85. Dalia T, Amr BS. *Pacemaker Indications*. StatPearls Publishing; 2020. http://www.ncbi.nlm.nih.gov/pubmed/29939600. Accessed January 12, 2021.

86. Berberian JG, Levine BJ, Brady WJ. *EMRA EKG Guide*. 1st ed. Dallas, TX: Emergency Medicine Residents' Association; 2017.

87. Salahuddin M, Cader F, Nasrin S, Chowdhury M. The pacemaker-twiddler's syndrome: An infrequent cause of pacemaker failure. *BMC Res Notes*. 2016;9(1):1-5. doi:10.1186/s13104-015-1818-0

88. Lesnick J, Cooper B, Doshi P. Twiddler's Syndrome. *Clin Pract Cases Emerg Med*. 2019;3(3):299-300. doi:10.5811/cpcem.2019.4.42123

89. Abu-haniyeh A, Hajouli S. *Pacemaker Mediated Tachycardia*. StatPearls Publishing; 2020. http://www.ncbi.nlm.nih.gov/pubmed/32809666. Accessed February 2, 2021.

90. Batehnb J, Gunderson T, Forfang K. Tachycardias Related to Atrial Synchronous Ventricular Pacing. *Pacing Clin Electrophysiol*. 1982;5(4):471-475. doi:10.1111/j.1540-8159.1982.tb02263.x

91. Den Dulk K, Lindemans F, Bar F, Wellens HJJ. Pacemaker Related Tachycardias. *Pacing Clin Electrophysiol*. 1982;5(4):476-485. doi:10.1111/j.1540-8159.1982.tb02264.x

92. Boehnert MT, Lovejoy FH. Value of the QRS duration versus the serum drug level in predicting seizures and ventricular arrhythmias after an acute overdose of tricyclic antidepressants. *N Engl J Med*. 1985;313(8):474-479. doi:10.1056/NEJM198508223130804

93. Gray A, Talari G, Mirrakhimov AE, Barbaryan A, Ayach T, Chadha R. The Role of Sodium Bicarbonate in the Management of Some Toxic Ingestions. *Int J Nephrol*. 2017;2017:1-8. doi:10.1155/2017/7831358

94. Kerr GW, Mcguye AC, Wilkie S. Tricyclic antidepressant overdose: a review. doi:10.1136/emj.18.4.236

Index

Made in the USA
Middletown, DE
13 March 2021

35166635R00115